THE HOLLYWOOD FACELIFT

Nola Rocco

Barclay House
New York

A BARCLAY TRADE PAPERBACK
Published by: Barclay House
A division of the Zinn Publishing Group
ZINN COMMUNICATIONS / NEW YORK

Produced in Cooperation with
Atchity Entertainment International (AEI)

Copyright © 1995 by Zinn Communications

All rights reserved. No part of this book may be reproduced or transmitted in any form or by any means, electronic or mechanical, including photocopying, recording , or by any information storage and retrieval system, without the written permission of the Publisher, except where permitted by law.

ISBN: 0-935016-32-5

Printed in the United States of America

Library of Congress Cataloging-in-Publication Data

Rocco, Nola. 1940–
    The Hollywood facelift : Facelifting, cosmetic surgery, and the new you / by Nola Rocco.
    p.   cm
    ISBN 0-935016-32-5 (pbk. : alk. paper)
    1. Facelift—Popular works. 2. Facelifts—Patients—Nutrition. 3. Rejuvination—Nutrition aspects
I. Title.
RD119.5.F33R63   1995
617.5'20592–dc20   95-47577
                                   CIP

Cartoons created by Nola Rocco.
Cartoons illustrated by Suraiya Daud.

This book is dedicated to:

Lynda • Chris • Mia • Alice • Yvonne • Sarah • Elaine • Collette • Eva • Shirley • Lisa • Ruth • Kim • Carolyn • Jacqueline • Seline • Peter • Gina • Salome • Sheri • John • Judith • Suzanne • Silva • Renate • Hildy • Bill • Anita • Martha • Roberta • Linda • Joseph • Barbara • Terry • Joanne • June • Rita • Julie • Jack • Denise • Norma • Arline • Evelyn • Maria • Gilbert • Vicki • Stan • Cindy • Doug • Desiree • Sheila • Leslie • Valery • Sy • Debra • Lynn • Dories • Raymond • Myrna • Adele • Sandra • Rachel • Joan • Brenda • Red • Carrie • Craig • Harriet • Neil • Olfet • Marylin • Said • Carolyn • Joan • Dorcy • Deenaz • Patricia • Louise • Beverly • Elouise • Meyera • Rosa • Joni • Sandy • Marissa • Isa • Jean • Bill • Madelyn • David • Toby • Lynne • Marie • Frankie • Camella • Pamela • Dorren • Gail • Dennis • Laverne • Rebecca • Susan • Margie • Bonnie • Pat • Patty • Stacey • Janet • Jennifer • Laurel • Margaret • Agnes • Mimi • Moussa • Penne • Donna • Yoshiko • Zee • Gigi • Paula • Kristina • Roma • Victoria • Maureen • Laurie • Julie • Iris • Gabby • Carrolyn • Helen • Alan • Jill • Martine • Nancy • Marjory • Marianne • Amelia • Carly • Roe Landa • Kay • Mildred • Candice • Dana • Walter • Daisy • Tootie • Bobbie • Lilly • Rosemary • Tiana • Felice • Sydney • Birdie • Thomas • Joe • Diane • Noorna • Janice • Debbra • Debra • Nahid • Vic • Marian • Nina • Kathy • Ben • Gretchen • Silvia • Eunice • Tisha • Daniel • Rhoda • Inger • Beth • Pete • Fern • Teran • Ester • Michelle • Lorna • Claudia • Dolores • Sue • Elenor • Helene • Gina • Dorothy • Jocelyn • Natalie • Cheri • Wilhelmina • Lorraine • Benji • Lavonne • Ada • Inge • Elizabeth • Patrick • Phillis • Francesco • Jim • Gabrielle • Jeff • Thelma • Betty • Flora • Mareta • Arthur • Hideko • Abigail • Rosaline • Karen • Kim • Olive • Eugene • Teresa • Bernardo • Julia • Geno • Sundri • Steven • Estela • Sally • Claire • Dorita • Peg • Mona • Chiko • Ella • Willa • Gladys • Grace • Lois • Angela • Gloria • Zelda • Kay • Wendy • Claudine • Joyce • Sharon • Eileen • Lana • Frantz • Melissa • Richard • Barry • Tim • Peaches • Erna • Dianna • Edith • Hortencia • Josephine • Janette • Marcie • Mark • Serene • Howard • Ruthe • Paul • Tina • Tiffani • Fauna • Neena • Deena • Anna Maria • Maxine • Annette • Emi • Al • Devon • Jocelyn • Gaylord • Estelle • Randi • Andrea • Gari • Marna • Gerry • Izumi • Tom • Genie • Marjorie • Neal • Idell • B.J. • Charlotte • September • Lee • Chris • James • Polly • Alyson • Virginia • Edward • Danai • Cathy • Doret • Hannah • Trinidad • Creig • Roseline • Marylee • Sobel • Hanna • Billy • Anne Shirley • Stella • Marina • Clide • Vera • Artetta • Rae • Michael • Persian • Adrianne • Kitti • Alisa • Judy • Colinette • Connie • Robin • Jack • Samantha • Yolanda

...and other Hidden Garden guests whose names are too well known that people just **might suspect.**

Thank you . . .

Teal, my daughter, for coming up with the perfect hideaway name: The Hidden Garden, and for your creative and delightful logo and art work. And, more importantly, for your patience, understanding and loving support. I love you.

and

Miriam Radstrom, R.N., expert in cosmetic surgery, who took the time to listen to my "idea" and whose personal encouragement and professional advice formed the concept and philosophy of The Hidden Garden.

and

The Staff, who not only have excellent professional skills but a sincere true love of people and who enjoy being at The Hidden Garden. It is this sense of understanding and caring that rings throughout our hideaway and is felt by our Guests. It's their wonderful attitude that makes The Hidden Garden a home away from home.

. . .**Thank you!**

Nola
The Hidden Garden Housemother

Introduction

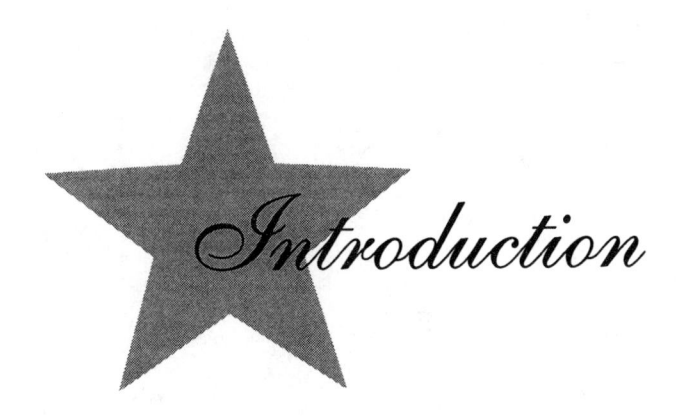

The Hidden Garden is a private hideaway in the heart of Beverly Hills, a unique, charming "Bed and Breakfast," with professional care. Guests come from all over the world to hide out after a cosmetic surgery procedure. Under the careful eye of our staff and the pleasant surroundings of *The Hidden Garden*, they re-enter the world rested, more attractive and rejuvenated.

The first part of the book, Part I, is designed to enlighten the lay person about cosmetic surgery in general on a basic level and to encourage the reader to seek the professional advice of a qualified, experienced plastic surgeon. It is not meant to be a scholarly effort to promote plastic surgery. *The Hidden Garden* does not promote or recommend any plastic surgeon or is it in any way connected with any plastic surgeon. It does provide post-operative care for patients of plastic surgeons in the Beverly Hills area and this excellent post-op care encourages the best results. It is this expertise for which *The Hidden Garden* is famous, and this book will share this information with you.

Part II, **The Hollywood Facelift Diet**, outlines specific day by day meals, a twenty-eight day gourmet menu to protect and help your new face as it heals. This diet is wonderful for anyone looking for a low fat, low sugar, no salt diet. You do not need a facelift to benefit from this diet.

Part III, **The Hidden Garden Cookbook**, is dedicated to a low calorie, low budget, easy to prepare, *and* incredibly delicious, "dinner party," Spa Cuisine! Our delicious Spa Cuisine is renowned among our guests, and because of their constant requests for our recipes, **The Hidden Garden Cookbook** was developed.

Nola

Table of Contents

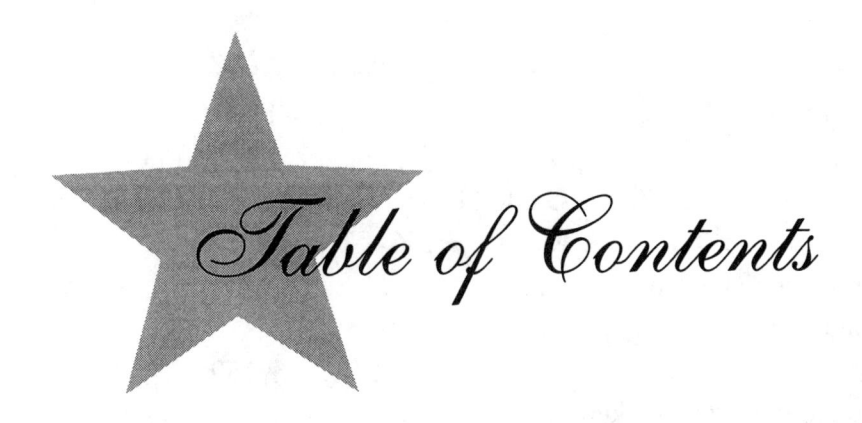

PART I

The Hollywood Facelift . . . . ★1
How To Prevent A Facelift . . . . ★3
The Big Decision . . . . ★7
A Facelift Is A Bargain! . . . . ★11
The Cost . . . . ★13
How To Select A Doctor . . . . ★15
What The Doctors Don't Tell You And
 What You Must tell The Doctor . . . . ★21
Looking Good: Count The Ways . . . . ★25
Husbands And Wives Do It . . . . ★51
For Men Only . . . . ★53
Face The Risk . . . . ★57
Be Prepared . . . . ★61
Hiding Out . . . . ★71
To Tell Or Not To Tell . . . . ★77
A Wrinkle In Time . . . . ★79
What's "Hot" In Beverly Hills . . . . ★85
The New You! . . . . ★89
What You Can Do To Hide An Old Look . . . . ★91
The Lighter Side . . . . ★95

PART II

The Hollywood Facelift Diet . . . . ★103
Introduction . . . . ★105

★ IX ★

PART III

The Hidden Garden Cookbook .... ★151
Salads .... ★153
    Fresh Romaine Lettuce With The Hidden Garden Pesto .... ★155
    Fresh Basil-Tomato Salad .... ★156
    The Hidden Garden Chopped Salad .... ★157
    Mint Cucumber Salad .... ★158
Soups .... ★159
    The Hidden Garden Homemade Chicken Soup .... ★161
    Country Inn Potato Leek Soup .... ★162
    Bay Shrimp Bisque .... ★163
    Fresh Tomato Mushroom Bisque .... ★164
    The Hidden Garden Homemade Carrot Soup .... ★165
    Broccoli Soup .... ★166
    Garden Fresh Chunky Vegetable Soup .... ★167
    Chilled Cantaloupe-Pineapple Soup .... ★168
Omelettes .... ★169
    Avocado and Cream Omelette .... ★171
    Mushroom Omelette .... ★172
    Spinach Omelette .... ★173
    Goat Cheese Omelette .... ★174
Fish .... ★175
    Broiled Chilean Sea Bass .... ★177
    Poached Norwegian Salmon .... ★178
    Bay Scallops .... ★179
    Nola's Scampi and Herbs .... ★180
Chicken .... ★181
    Chicken Picatta with Fresh Garden Herbs .... ★183
    Baked Cornish Game Hens .... ★184
Pasta .... ★185
    The Hidden Garden Homemade Manicotti .... ★187
    The Hidden Garden Pasta with Pesto .... ★188
    Special Italian Rigatoni Noodles .... ★189
    Grandma Rocco's Pasta Primavera .... ★190
Polenta .... ★191
    The "Real" Italian Country Style Polenta .... ★193

Table Of Contents

Wild Rice .... ★195
    Wild Wild rice .... ★197
Veggies .... ★199
    Baked or grilled Japanese Eggplant .... ★201
    Baked Scallopini Squash .... ★202
    Steamed zucchini with Fresh Basil .... ★203
Tea Bread and Muffins .... ★205
    Banana-Fruit Tea Bread .... ★207
    Grandmother's Oat bran Mini Muffins .... ★208
Cakes and Pies .... ★209
    Zangy Lemon Poppy Seed Cake .... ★211
    Nola's 4th of July Apple Pie .... ★212
    Nola's Incredible Blueberry Pie .... ★213
    Pear Tart .... ★214
    Pie pastry .... ★215
Milkshakes .... ★217
    Blueberry Milkshake .... ★219
    Strawberry-Banana Milkshake .... ★220
    Dr. Frisher's Shake .... ★221
    Chocolate Milkshake .... ★222
    Diane's Fruit Smoothie .... ★223
Chocolates .... ★225
    Teal's Chocolate-Chocolate-Chocolate Chip Cake .... ★227
    Extra Dark Chocolate brownies .... ★228
    Heavenly Chocolate Mousse with Creme Fraiche .... ★229
Desserts and Sweet Sauces .... ★231
    Poached Pears with Cinnamon Sticks .... ★233
    Mother's Egg Custard .... ★234
    Poached Prunes and Apricot Compote .... ★235
    Yummy Tapioca Pudding .... ★236
    Custard Sauce .... ★237
    Creme Fraiche .... ★238

Foot Notes .... ★239

The Hollywood Facelift

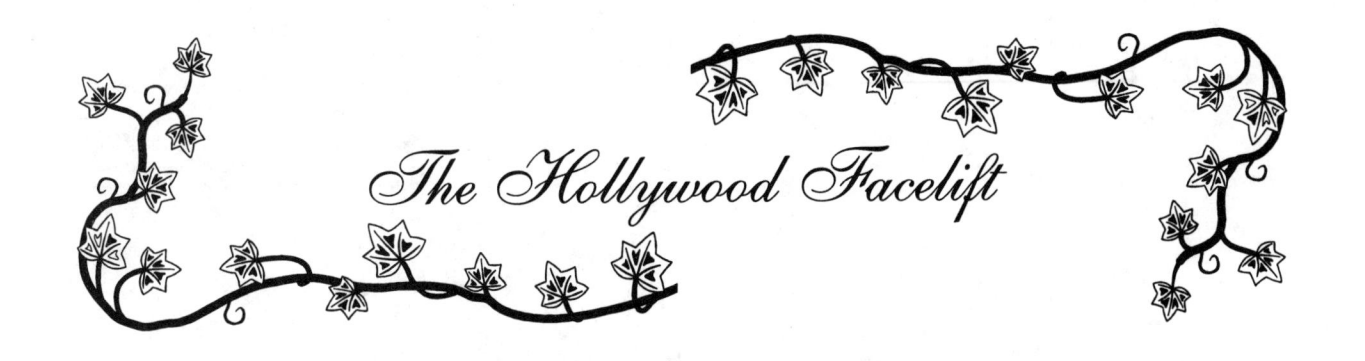

Part 1

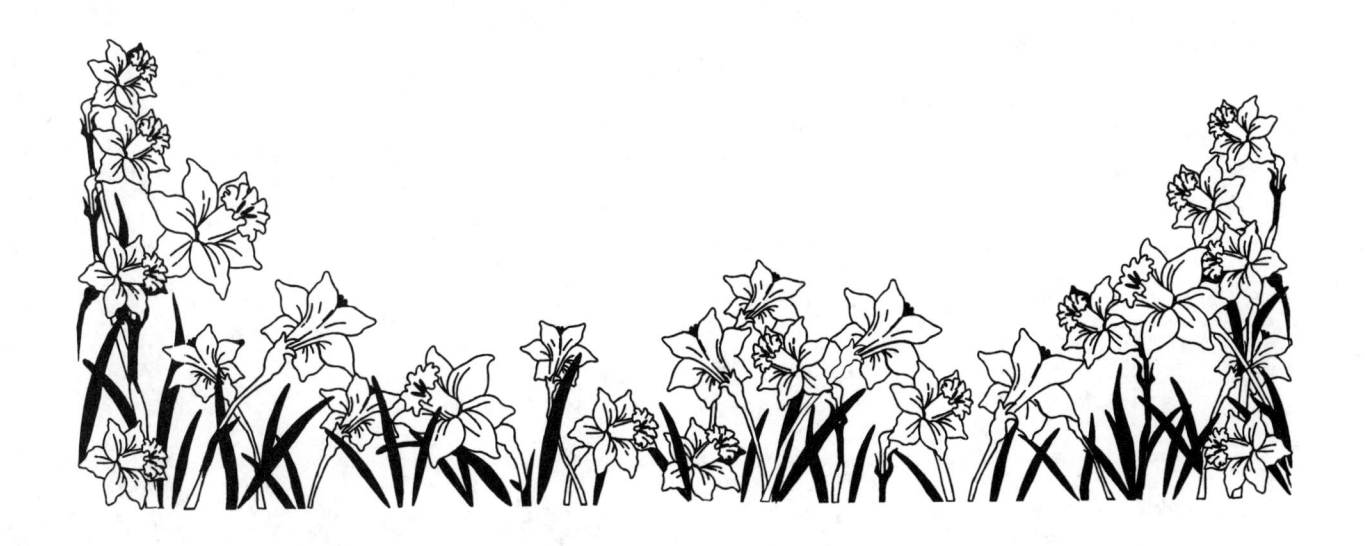

How To Prevent A Facelift

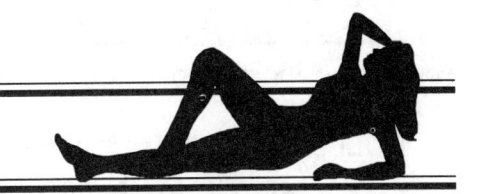

Some people are blessed with a marvelous inherited bone structure, an absolutely perfect nose, incredibly gorgeous eyes and a perfect peaches and cream complexion. We are constantly bombarded with perfect bodies modeling in the fashion magazines. And each time we see a gorgeous model, our own face becomes more "awful."

Cosmetic companies have continuous advertising campaigns for their latest skin rejuvenator. Retin-A is called a miracle drug, and Collagen is the non-surgical facelift. These products and drugs have their place, but they are only temporary.

Is it possible to prevent a facelift? Why do some people need a facelift before others?

Yes, it is possible to prevent a facelift if you follow just a few simple rules. But you must follow them all and you must follow them **all your life, starting at an early age**.

RULE #1: *SLEEP ON YOUR BACK.* Sleeping on your face stretches and creases the skin.

RULE #2: *AVOID YO-YO DIETING.* The first place we lose weight or gain weight is in the face. With time, our skin no longer "springs" back, the loss of fat beneath the skin leaves it "sagging" especially in the jowl area. While younger skin can take more "Yo-yo"ing, as we age, the effects of gaining and losing weight will show in loss of muscle tone. It is best to find a good, comfortable, healthy weight and maintain it. Since our bodies seem to gain weight as we age, rather than dieting it's more advantageous to just eat a little less and change some eating habits, for example, substitute skim milk for whole milk, frozen non-fat yogurt for ice cream. On the average people gain one pound per year starting at age thirty even if they don't eat one calorie more! Therefore by age forty we are ten pounds heavier. And, we wonder where it came from?

Do not stuff yourself. Snacking five or six times a day on healthy foods is better than one large dinner at night. You will burn off the snacks you eat throughout the day, leaving nothing to be stored as fat. Your diet should include adequate amounts of potassium, Vitamin C with Bioflavonoids and a good multiple Vitamin. Eat healthy foods, high in carbohydrates, protein and fiber and low in fats.

RULE #3: *EXERCISE REGULARLY.* Need we say more? Exercise brings oxygen to the blood vessels. Oxygen is an anti-aging agent and it's free!

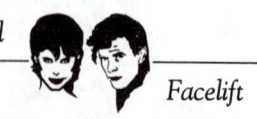

RULE #4. *LIMIT YOUR INTAKE OF COFFEE AND ALCOHOL.* Coffee (caffeine) and alcohol raise blood pressure and dehydrate the body. Dehydration causes the skin to wrinkle. Limit your coffee and alcohol to no more than two drinks each per day.

RULE #5: *DRINK LOTS OF WATER.* Drink at least eight glasses per day. Water cleanses the body and is necessary to replenish the water lost from exercise, alcohol, smoking, and caffeine consumption. It is common sense; if you are dehydrated, your skin is going to show wrinkles and water is necessary to "plump" out your skin. A prune is a plum without water!

RULE #6. *SLEEP WITH CLEAN SKIN.* After you have carefully washed off all make-up and daily "dirt," avoiding soaps that are alkaline, *lightly* apply moisturizer on to *warm, wet* skin, especially at night. It is important that you choose the right moisturizer for your skin type and that your skin be clean so it can breathe. Never rub your face hard when applying anything. Even rubbing with "upward" motion is bad if you are pulling and stretching your skin.

RULE #7: *STAY OUT OF THE SUN.* The sun is extremely damaging to the skin. Sun destroys the collagen enzymes and changes the skin texture which causes pre-mature aging. Use sunblock even when riding in a car. The sun's harmful rays bounce off the hood of the car, through the windshield and windows to those inside. Snow, ice, sand and concrete reflect the sun's rays. It is necessary to apply a sunscreen year round and reapply every three to four hours if you are outside. It also helps to wear a broad-brimmed hat when you are outside between the hours of 10 A.M. to 3 P.M. Wear sunglasses to protect your eyes and prevent squinting.

RULE #8: *DON'T SMOKE.* Heavy smokers are many times more likely to have wrinkles than nonsmokers. The muscle action of the lips causes wrinkles above the lip. Not only do smokers have many more lines on their faces as they grow older, but the skin texture loses its elasticity, sooner. Nicotine in the bloodstream causes the blood vessels to constrict, depriving the skin of a full nourishing blood supply.

RULE #9. *KEEP ORCHIDS IN YOUR BEDROOM.* Typical house plants give off oxygen in the daytime but orchids give off oxygen at *night*. It is rumored that Michael Jackson sleeps in a special room where fresh oxygen is circulated. Regular oxygen therapy treatments are believed to prevent aging.

RULE #10. *AVOID BROAD FACIAL EXPRESSIONS AND THE GNAWING OF FOOD.* Avoid eating large nuts and seeds, crusty breads or any foods like Beef Jerky or chewy caramel candy that requires your mouth to be opened wide or for your teeth to grind for a long period. Do not chew gum!

A guest at the Hidden Garden had "one half" a facelift. Some fifteen or sixteen years prior to her facial surgery she had been in an automobile accident and was left partially paralyzed on the right side of her face. She had regained only partial muscle action of that paralyzed side. Because of the lack of full expressions on the right side of her face, she never developed any signs of aging on that side. Her other side, however, had aged over the years and developed sagging jowls and large wrinkles. Our guest had a facelift so that her aging side of her face would look like her non-aging side.

It is believed that exercising the facial muscles may cause wrinkles and expression lines, and be especially aware of those forehead *"thinking"* lines. Animated people, TV personalities and performers, have a tendency to need facial cosmetic surgery sooner. Joan Rivers and Carol Burnett types are facelift candidates. Many stars have had "nips and tucks" for years just for that reason. On the other hand, Aida Grey, at eighty plus looked incredible and had never had a facelift. But she always maintained gorgeous skin and soft facial expressions.

Over the years, yawning, coughing, sneezing cause wrinkles. Both smiling and kissing can cause wrinkles and facial expression lines as well! And of course so does talking.

Nola's Note: To avoid facial wrinkles, grit your teeth together while speaking. Try it!

There you have it. Ten rules to avoid a facelift. If you can live by them, more power to you. If you can't, read on!

Sometimes, without knowing it, our own personality and lifestyle can cause a facelift.

The Big Decision

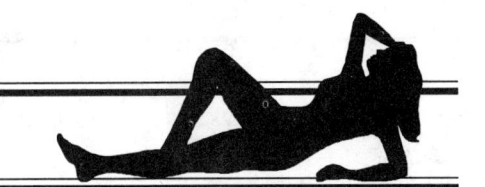

Plastic surgery has become a more common and acceptable experience as our society, our jobs and, we, ourselves demand to look good. Years ago, men and women had their weekly hair and nail appointments. Today, we can add to that ritual a facial, pedicure, leg waxing, lash tinting, hair weaving, and skin bleaching. And, more recently, men and women include on their beauty ritual injectable collagen, a facial skin peel, fat injection, and of course the yearly visit to their plastic surgeon for a little "nip and tuck" here and there.

Younger and younger people are considering cosmetic surgery. With career women playing a stronger role in society they see how quickly and painlessly they can take "years" off an aging look.

Although we have had a few "Plastic Surgery junkies" at The Hidden Garden, most of our guests agree that they have elected surgery after much thought. Just when did they decide . . .

"When I woke up one morning and noticed that I looked like my mother." (F, 47, face/eyes)

"Started looking at other women instead of men ... asking if I look as good as she looks." (F, 51, face/eyes)

"Tried every haircut and every hair color, nothing worked ..." (F, 56, face/eyes/browlift)

"My ex-husband offered it to me as part of a divorce settlement ... later I realized he thought that he'd be ahead of the game if I looked younger, I would remarry sooner ... less spousal support he'd have to pay." (F, 48, face/eyes)

Nola's Note: The ex-husband went in for a facelift a year later.

"I'm on this soap, you see, and my character doesn't grow old as fast as I do in real life ... I have a look to maintain." (M, 46, face)

"It first started with my eyes, that was four years ago, then I noticed lines around my lip — but when I *really* looked at myself, I noticed lines all over!" (F, 52, face/eyes)

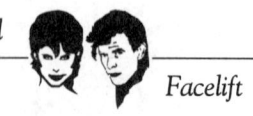

"No question about the face ... it was the *nose* that I couldn't make up my mind about ... my nose is me, I couldn't do the nose. At 62 — why? It's too obvious!" (F, 62, face/eyes)

"Looking at myself in the mirror ... I looked great ... but then I put my glasses on ...." (F, 43, face/eyes)

"My husband got a new Secretary ..." (F, 47, face/eyes and breast augmentation)

"My wife spent too many hours with her Tennis instructor ..." (M. 55, face/eyes)

"Cost of Collagen was killing me!" (F, 54, face/eyes/peel)

"I've worked out for four years, every muscle in my body is tight ... except my gut ... couldn't seem to get that trim waistline ... Lipo was the only way to get rid of that roll." (M, 42, Liposuction)

"Started a new life ... my ex ran off with this twenty-two year old bimbo. Kids think she's gorgeous. Well, they are right, she is. I know I can't be gorgeous. I just want to look good. I want my kids to be proud of me." (F, 42, face/eyes/browlift)

"We just want to look as good as we feel ... Friends think we're on a trip ... we are!" (Husband and wife, 55 and 53, face/eyes)

"Those 'yuppies' are coming on stronger at the Board Meetings, been with the company for twenty-seven years and no one listens to me anymore ... I needed a refreshed look. Don't want to look younger, just don't want to look tired." (M, 60, face/eyes)

"I got a ten million dollar house in Santa Barbara and the cutest twenty-eight year old girlfriend. I know I'll keep the house, but I'm not so sure I'll be able to keep the girl." (M, 65, face/eyes/brow)

"It's really incredible how one can change a body. This is my eighth cosmetic surgery within a year. I know you are calling me a 'P.S. junkie', but ... why not? I have the health, the money and the time and I am obsessed with the idea of a perfect body." (M, 42, butt tuck)

"It's cheaper than a shrink ... all my divorced girlfriends are spending fortunes on therapy." (F, 52, facelift)

"I cut to the chase ... He left me for a thirty-two year old. If I can look forty-two and grab a thirty-two year old ... we'll be even!" (F, 52, face, eyes, lipo, breast lift and augmentation)

"Six months is my son's wedding. I don't want to look like the ex-wife. I want to look like an energetic, which I am — friendly, which I am, — attractive, which I am not! — mother. Lunching with my girlfriends, I look good. But when I lunch with the ex, I look old. I don't feel old ... I'm happy with the divorce. I just want my son to be proud of me and I want to be proud of me, too. I want to look the best I can." (F, 56, face/eyes/forehead)

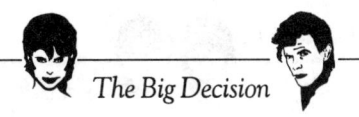

"Twenty-two years of sun and sailing ... it's killed my face! All I expect is to look my age. And if I look better, that's great too." (F, 55, face/eyes/peel)

"I can't beat 'time' but I'm sure going to try to keep just one step ahead ...." (F, 42, face/eyes)

"Just want to look as good as I feel. When my face looked older than what I felt ... it was time to balance the act ...." (F, 49, face/eyes/brow)

"My book publisher needed pictures. Jowls appeared. Pictures don't lie!" (F, 55, face/eyes)

"There is absolutely no way I'm going to look old. I feel thirty-five, I have the body of a thirty-five year old and I'll be damned to look older than I feel. Best of all, with a facelift, I can look thirty-five yet have the experience of my age ... now can you beat that!" (F, 49, face/eyes/nose)

"I'm fifty and treated myself to a new face. The best investment I can make is in me!" (F, 50, face/eyes/breast)

"My girlfriend took this fancy, jet-set singles cruise, a ten day vacation, $5,000. She wanted me to go along. I took my own cruise ... $10,000, ten years younger! Who got the better deal?" (F, 47, face/eyes)

"My husband is very upset ... but I want to look good. It's important to me." (F, 65, face/eyes)

"My girls have been after me to do this for three years now. 'You put us through college, Mom ... now it's time to do something for yourself.'" (F, 57, face/eyes)

"I'm not going to wait 'till I'm fifty, or forty, or even thirty. I want to look as good as I can, now, and enjoy it." (F, 23, eyes/nose/chin/cheek/breast/lipo of abdominal area and thighs)

"It was my birthday. My husband offered me either a cruise or a facelift. I chose the facelift! I can have a cruise anytime!" (F, 53, face/eyes/nose/cheek)

"I have several younger boyfriends. With a fresh looking face I think I can get a few more!" (F, 68, face, eyes, chin, nose)

"I've been courting this girl for several years and I'm not getting anywhere with her. I'm a businessman, a successful one, with nice cars, a boat at the Marina, cabin at Lake Tahoe. I have everything but a young face ...." (M, 53, facelift)

"We're going to have our fortieth Wedding Anniversary next month. I'm giving my husband a new body. I said to my husband when I went into surgery this morning, 'Hubby, kiss these ol' titties good-by!'" (F, 56, breasts, lipo)

"I kept looking at my face. I'm only thirty-three, an artist, but something was wrong. When my doctor suggested the browlift ... that was it!" (F, 33, brow)

"When I refinanced, the loan officer asked if I was using the money to remodel. I sure did. I scheduled a facelift!" (F, 49, face, eyes, forehead)

"After twenty years my sister paid back the money I loaned her. I never thought I'd ever see that money again. It was found money!" (F, 50, face, eyes/nose/forehead)

"I treated myself to a fiftieth birthday present!" (F, 49½, face/eyes/forehead)

"My sister wanted this more than me, but when I thought about it more seriously, I realized 'we' had to do it together." (Twins, F, age 50, face/eyes/forehead)

Nola's Note: They still look alike, but ten years younger!

"Better take advantage of what Mother Nature gave us before Father Time takes it away ..." (F, 69, face/eyes)

A Facelift Is A Bargain

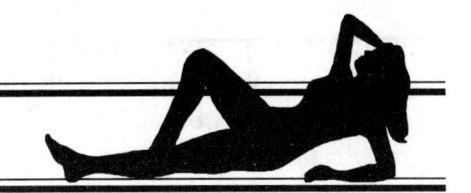

People spend fortunes on haircuts, hair color, cosmetics, trainers, gym memberships, health spas, beauty spas, clothes, diets, Club Med weekends, exercise equipment, creams, cruises, laxatives and therapists. Their goal is to look good, look young, maintain a healthy image, all, in reality, to fight aging. *And why not!* People who keep in shape, exercise, eat cautiously, who want to maintain a younger image, usually care about themselves. They believe in themselves. They see it as their number one investment. Cosmetic Surgery is an investment opportunity. Unlike ten years ago when only the rich and famous TV personalities and movie stars considered it, career people, both single and married, women and men see it as part of "keeping fit," looking as good as they can, no matter the costs.

Think about it. A facelift can take ten years off one's appearance. If you were to amortize the cost of the surgery over ten years, you'd be surprised how *inexpensive* it is to have cosmetic surgery.

The cost of a facelift in the Beverly Hills area would run between $8,000-$12,000. An average cost of $10,000 over a 10-year time comes to $1,000 per year or $83.33 per month. Most women and even men spend at least that on monthly hair needs, manicures, even cosmetics that often do not achieve what a facelift does, and yet people continue to spend fortunes month after month trying desperately, searching for a way to look younger. **A facelift is a BARGAIN!**

Combining several facial procedures at the same time does save money. The most common are face and eyes. Adding a nose or cheek implant or chin implant is probably the most one would want to do at one time. Usually by the mid-forties and early fifties, you would need at least a facelift and eyelift. Often doing just the face will only accentuate tired looking eyes, which will take you back into surgery. Having several procedures done simultaneously is not only less expensive, it usually takes the same amount of recovery time. And even more important, the result is incredible.

I never ask, but, a male guest at The Hidden Garden shared his costs with me.

Surgeon's Fee:	Face	$8,000	Anesthesiologist	$1,200
	Eyes	$4,000	Operating Room	$1,200
	Nose	$6,000	Other	$ 600

TOTAL: $21,000.00

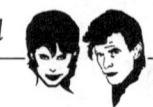

However, because of combining the head procedures, he told me that he saved money. Individually, it would have been closer to $27,000, a $6,000 savings!

Many men would rather have the "self-investment" of $20,000 rather than a Porsche or BMW. And, again, amortize that $20,000 over many years of enjoyment and "looking good." *If you add the financial rewards of job advancement and social contacts, the surgery pays for itself within a year or two.*

A complete new face and breast augmentation can cost $25,000 to $43,000.

Probably the most expensive day of your life! But it could be well worth it. A darling young lady in her early twenties not only had her double chin removed but added an eye lift, a nose job, cheek implants, chin implants, breast augmentation and liposuction (fat removal) of her thighs and waistline. She had both a new face *and* a new body. (Eight hours of surgery by two doctors.) She decided that she wasn't going to wait until she turned fifty, she was going to enjoy her new look all her young life. Another young woman, a college graduate, chose breast augmentation over a Cartier watch.

There is definitely a financial advantage as well as the savings of time when combining several procedures, if your doctor feels comfortable about doing so. You avoid repeating the risks and trauma to your body twice. *Certain combinations or procedures work well together; others need to be considered very seriously.*

The most common combinations are the full facelift (face and neck), eyelift (uppers and lowers) and a browlift. In many cases, if you don't do the eyes with the face, the eyes will look very tired against the new face. Also popular is adding a peel to smooth out the fine lines of the upper lip and eye area. The healing time is the same.

Based on the fact that you are healthy, have passed all your pre-op tests, and are under the care of a Board Certified Surgeon experienced in the procedures, there is little danger.

Combining two surgical procedures, only one being cosmetic, can save time and costs. A hysterectomy with tummy tuck (abdominoplasty) is not uncommon, or a hernia repair and a tummy tuck.

When considering combinations of procedures, it is most important that you get several consultations from Board Certified Surgeons and because each case must be considered individually, taking into account age, health, previous surgeries, and lifestyles. *Too many procedures at once can over-traumatize the body.* Most doctors will not do long surgeries. They want their work to be the best. The average facelift with eyes takes three to four hours. Most doctors will not take the unnecessary risks involved in a surgery that lasts over six hours.

Many surgeons have a time limit as to how long they feel comfortable a person should be under a general anaesthesia and how long the surgeon feels he can perform. Six hours of surgery is about maximum. Most doctors like to keep it under 5 hours. All surgeries must be skillfully and carefully done. You can't rush an artist. Incredible when you think about it.

Mothers, please note: Don't just encourage your son to be a doctor, encourage him to be a Plastic Surgeon!

The Cost

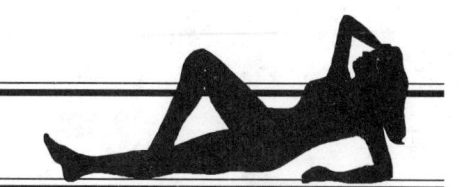

Location: Beverly Hills   Year: 1995

	Surgeon's Fee	Operating Room	Anesthesiologist
Facelift	$6,000 -12,000	$ 800 -1,000	$ 800 -1,000
Eyes	$3,000 - 6,000	$ 500 -1,000	$ 800 -1,000
Nose	$3,500 - 9,000	$ 700 -1,000	$ 700 -1,000
Chin Augmentation	$2,500 - 3,000	$ 500 - 800	$ 450 - 600
Cheek Augmentation	$2,500 - 3,000	$ 500 - 800	$ 450 - 600
Hair Flap	$5,000 (varies with needs)		
Liposuction	$ 500 - 8,000		
Chemical Peel	$ 500 - 5,000 (varies with needs)		
Dermabrasion	$ 500 - 5,000 (varies with needs)		
Breast Reduction	$4,500 - 6,000	$ 500 -1,000	$ 600 - 800
Breast Augmentation	$3,000 - 6,000	$ 500 -1,000	$ 600 - 800
Breast Lift	$3,000 - 6,000	$ 500 -1,000	$ 600 - 800
Tummy Tuck	$4,000 - 6,000	$1,000 -1,600	$ 650 -1,000

COMBOS

Face and eyes	$ 6,000 -11,500	± $2,050	± $975
Forehead, face, eyes	$ 9,500 -14,000	± $1,950	± $925
Face, eyes, nose	$13,000 -20,000	± $2,050	± $975
Cheek/Chin	$ 4,500 - 6,000	± $1,250	± $600
Breast Lift/Augmentation	$ 7,500 - 9,000	± $2,650	± $750

Consultation fee: $75 - $500. Sometimes applied to the Surgery cost, sometimes not.

How To Select A Doctor

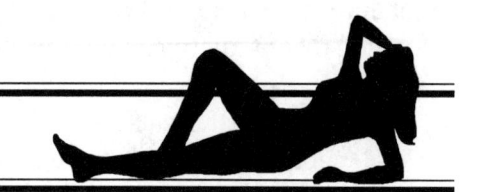

You can't select a plastic surgeon like going on a date.

You can't judge him on his clothes (they all wear white coats).

You can't evaluate his surgical skills by the car he drives.

Just for fun, how about a little bit of Beverly Hills "gossip," guess who drives what!

Michael Churukian	Porsche	Lawrence Koplin	Porsche
Alfred Cohen	XJS	Robert Kotler	Checker Cab
Garth Fisher	SL 600 MBZ Convertible	Lawrence Lefkoff	BMW Convertible
Richard Fleming	Porsche/Rolls Royce	Malcolm Lesavoy	Prefers: Missouri Trotters
Stephen Genender	MBZ Convertible	Bernard Markowitz	Porsche Cabriolet
Harry Glassman	Bentley	Toby Mayer	Prefers: Polo Ponies
Barbara Hayden	Volvo	Timothy Miller	Lexus
Steven Hoefflin	Blazer/Porsche Carrera	Jon Perlman	Jeep/MBZ/Jaguar/Classic Rolls Royce
David Hopp	Mercedes	Frank Ryan	BMW
Robert Hutcherson	Porsche Turbo	Lawrence Seifert	Jeep/Porsche/Bicycles
Raj Kanodia	Ferrari	Gary Tearston	Saab Convertible
Henry Kawamoto	Jaguar/Chauffeured Limo	John Williams	Lexus
Brian Kinney	BMW	Robin Yuan	350 SL MBZ
T. Gregory Kirianoff	Rolls Royce	Harvey Zarem	Mercedes

Nola's Note: Doctors not listed: their cars are already public knowledge!

Now, let's get serious!!!

You can't believe rumors or accept someone else's choice or opinion. You can make a good selection by being observant and asking some very important basic questions.

ASK: Is he Board Certified?

The word "Plastic" comes from the Greek word "Plastikos" which means to mold or give form. Plastic Surgery is a specialty that makes it possible to do just that - mold and re-form the human body.

Procedures that heal and restore patients with disfigurement from injury, disease, or birth defect are called reconstructive. These include surgical correction of deformities caused by the following:

- cleft lip and palate, ear deformities and other birth defects;
- abnormal growth or alignment of the jaw;
- burns, lacerations and other injuries from automobiles, home and work-related accidents;
- cancer, arthritis and other diseases.

Procedures that enhance appearance by recontouring facial and body features are called aesthetic or cosmetic. Cosmetic procedures include those that:

- minimize the effects of aging (including facelifts, eyelid surgery, chemical peels, dermabrasion and hair transplants);
- redefine undesirable facial features (including surgery on the nose, ears and chin);
- resculpt other body contours through fat reduction (liposuction),
- abdominoplasty ("tummy tuck"), and breast augmentation or lift or reduction.

Only two Boards certify their Surgeons to perform plastic surgery:

"Check for certification by the *American Board of Plastic Surgery*. American Board of Plastic Surgery (ABPS) certification means that the surgeon has completed undergraduate college, medical school, an approved surgery residency of at least three years, and an approved plastic surgery residency of an additional two to three years. Board certification then is obtained only after the candidate passes rigorous written and oral examinations administered by trained and experienced plastic surgeons.

"Remember—in most states, it is legal for any physician who holds a medical license, with or without surgical training, to call themselves a plastic or cosmetic surgeon. That's why understanding board certification is so important for the prospective patient.

"If there is confusion about a surgeon's board certification, you may consult the ABMS Compendium of Certified Medical Specialists or The Directory of Medical Specialists available at most libraries.

"Check for membership in the American Society of Plastic and Reconstructive Surgeons (ASPRS) or The American Society for Aesthetic Plastic Surgery (ASAPS). All members of these professional societies are certified by the American Board of Plastic Surgery. ASPRS represents the full scope of plastic surgery (reconstructive and aesthetic). Members of ASAPS are also trained as complete plastic surgeons but choose to concentrate their practice primarily in aesthetic surgery."[1]

These members are truly qualified to work on your whole body—head to toe.

The American Academy of Facial Plastic and Reconstructive Surgeons (AAFPRS) is composed of physicians performing cosmetic and reconstructive surgery of the face, head and neck.

"Facial plastic surgeons specialize in performing cosmetic and reconstructive surgery on the face, head, and neck region. As a group, facial plastic surgeons, who, for the most part are board certified in otolaryngology—head and neck surgery, do a major share of all facial plastic surgery performed in the United States."

"The American Academy of Facial Plastic and Reconstructive Surgery, Inc. (AAFPRS), is the world's largest association of facial plastic surgeons— those physicians performing cosmetic and reconstructive surgery of the face, head and neck. The Academy's bylaws provide that AAFPRS fellows be board-certified surgeons with training and experience in facial plastic surgery and be fellows of the American College of Surgeons."[2]

Nola's Note: I refer to doctors as being male but please note that there are female plastic surgeons who are very well qualified and do excellent work with fantastic results.

Don't waste your time with other organizations. Some are started by doctors with little guidelines and others are just local groups of doctors. Don't be impressed by the number of plaques a doctor has on his wall.

Because plastic surgery is profitable many doctors call themselves plastic surgeons and do plastic surgical procedures. *It is not illegal.* A qualified doctor will not hesitate to tell you his background and training.

ASK: What hospital is he associated with?

If it's some small unknown hospital — move on.

ASK: Who did he train with? Is the doctor associated with a Medical School. Does he teach or give seminars? Does he attend the yearly conventions?

A doctor can be young and very good if he has completed a *fellowship program* under a "Master" surgeon and gets to participate in many other surgeries before starting out on his own. For example, the plastic surgery fellowship program at UCLA is very, very selective of its doctors. Thousands of excellent doctors apply, but only a few are chosen. This training is the best. Doctors not only need to be certified and experienced but they also need to be up on the *latest procedures* and methods of surgery.

ASK: Exactly where will the sutures be? You need to know what to expect, where the scars will be. Facelift sutures in front of the ears are used on men but only sometimes on women. Sutures can leave a scar in front of the ear on the side of the face. Although buried in a man's beard, this scar can be obvious when a woman wears her hair back. (However, not a problem if you have a good surgeon.)

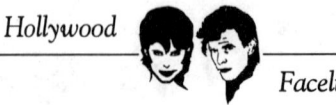

OBSERVE: Does the doctor care about himself? Is the doctor into health and beauty? Unlike other doctors, Plastic Surgeons are into looking good and keeping in shape. Does he play tennis, bicycle, golf, run, ski ... work out? A healthy, strong doctor allows himself the strength to perform long hours of surgery. You don't want a tired doctor working on your body! A facelift can take three to four concentrated hours of surgical skills.

OBSERVE: Does the doctor have an aesthetic sense? Look at the reception room? It is the first impression you get. Clean? Neat? Uncluttered? Restful?
Do the Post-Op patients run into the Pre-Op patients or are there private entrances? Private consultation times? Is the office organized? Are the Office Manager and Receptionist organized, friendly, happy to be there? Is there adequate staff? (One nurse cannot be the OR Tech and the Recovery Nurse and the secretary.) Excessive overhead is not something you want to pay for, but you need evidence of success. Whether a large or small office, be aware of cleanliness. Many surgeries are done in the office and it is important that the doctor has an updated OR (operating room) with all necessary emergency equipment or a state *approved* and licensed "Surgical Center."

OBSERVE: What is his attitude about himself and toward his work? Does he love what he is doing or would he rather be at the beach! Is his family life together? A doctor who is going through a divorce could be very ecstatic or very angry. Doctors are people.

A guest told me that one of her first questions to the consulting doctor was, "How's your sex life?" She was very serious. She chose a doctor who was in a happy relationship. "I felt like he would arrive to an early morning surgery contented."

ASK: Does he do magic? A guest fell in love with her doctor when he pulled out a little red ball from behind her ear. Turned out he did magic with the kids at the "burn" ward at a local children's hospital. Magician hands are very delicate and agile, swift and precise ... a good indication of a good surgeon.

ASK: To see and feel breast implants. You should not be led into the easiest surgical choice. Ask about the differences in various implant manufacturers' designs. The new implant versus the old. (Improved saline implants are now available.)

ASK: Where the implant will be inserted:

With breast implants: Under the arm? Under the muscle? Through the nipple?

With cheek implants: Insertion through the mouth or under the eyelid?

With chin implants: Insertion through the mouth or under the chin?

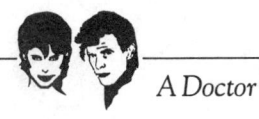

ASK: What are the risks? Remember, although plastic surgery procedures are normally safe, the unexpected can happen. In addition, medicine is an inexact science and results are sometimes unpredictable. The doctor should discuss the risks with you. If he doesn't, select another doctor. The broader your surgeon's training and experience, the greater your chances for a satisfactory result. It is most important that you feel 100% comfortable with your doctor. After all, it is your elective surgery and it takes "two to tango"—a skilled plastic surgeon and a healthy patient. The two well-matched present a wonderful result.

OBSERVE: Is the plastic surgeon sensitive? He must help you decide whether plastic surgery is right for you—physically and emotionally. Patients who expect the surgery to solve their social, sexual or business difficulties are disappointed if they find these problems still exist after the operation. In addition, patients who want a procedure that is unrealistic in view of their particular body structure are also doomed to disappointment. Or a woman who was never "beautiful" can't expect a facelift to make her so, it will make her look younger and better. Open discussion with a surgeon who is knowledgeable and sensitive to these problems—and who won't make promises that may not be kept—will help assure a happy outcome, a good result.

A good result is "a happy well motivated patient who seeks to improve him or herself and not change the world ... children and adolescents have a belief that if they change their appearance they significantly alter the world around them ... a magical wish."[3]

What The Doctors Don't Tell You And What You Must Tell The Doctor

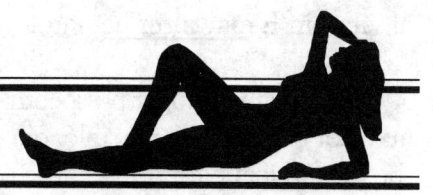

Honesty is the most important factor in establishing a strong, positive relationship. And it is equally true during your consultation with the plastic surgeon. You need to discuss your motivations and expectations and the surgeon must discuss the possible risks and variations in outcome. This dialogue is very important for a good "result."

Be aware that looking at a doctor's before and after pictures of some other client is not you. Be aware that computer imaging is only an estimate of a look. No guarantees! Taking in magazine pictures of some gorgeous model with a beautiful face, a perfect nose, and incredible eyes can help a doctor get a feeling for what you like, but in most cases those magazine pictures will be far from what belongs on your face. We all have dreams, but one has to be realistic.

Doctors discuss the recovery time rather quickly. This is a time when you must take care to be gentle with yourself. Doctors often don't tell you exactly what you can do and what you can't. If you have limited days to be "hiding out," be sure the doctor gives you a realistic picture of what to expect so you can plan accordingly.

Doctors will remind their pre-operative patients not to take aspirin two to three weeks before surgery. But they often forget to remind the patient to abstain from other products that contain aspirin, like Pepto-Bismol and Ben Gay.

Vitamin E is another tricky substance seldom mentioned. Michael Churukian, M.D., F.A.C.S., Camden Surgery Center in Beverly Hills, did a study on vitamin E. Churukian's research report states:

"Vitamin E refers to a group of fat-soluble substances found in certain plants. The biologically active substance is alpha-D-tocopherol and it serves mainly as an antioxidant. About 25% to 50% of an oral dose is absorbed and eighty percent is metabolized by the liver in one week. Vitamin E has been heavily promoted in the popular press for myriad qualities including the reversal of the aging process. Whereas the minimum daily requirement is 8 to 10 i.u., megadoses from 100 to 1600 i.u.

daily are taken by approximately 13% of the American population. ...[E]vidence that high doses of vitamin E may alter hematologic parameters comes from several different lines of work...

"Although a proper prospective study of the effect of Vitamin E on hemostasis in surgical wounds may not be ethically possible, our retrospective study suggests that vitamin E is contra-indicated in the presurgical patient. Because of the long half-life of this fat-soluble vitamin, patients should abstain from usage for at least two weeks pre-operatively."

Papaya has been questioned as well. (Papaya is used in meat tenderizing.) Cases have been reported that large doses of papaya tablets as well as eating and drinking papaya juices can cause bleeding after surgery. Papaya, wonderful for healing, should be avoided immediately after surgery and ten days to two weeks before surgeries, just to be on the safe side. (See: Be Prepared)

Two extremes of personalities seem to emerge when it comes to having cosmetic surgery. The conservative client who wants to look "better," 5-10 years younger, (i.e. Ivana Trump) and the client who wants to look more beautiful, attractive, who wants to bury the old look for a "new look" (i.e. Michael Jackson).

Whatever the look you want, you must express this at the time of consultation, otherwise you will not get the result you want and you will be disappointed. Take a tape recorder and record the consultation.

One of the Hidden Garden's favorite guests, Steve C. from Fresno, California, made a wonderful suggestion. "Go to a professional photographer late in the afternoon, when you are most tired, and take your own 'before' pictures." In this way, both you and the doctor can discuss the areas that are of concern. Mark up the photos. Bring these with you to surgery so the doctor will not forget the little areas of concern. Once you are asleep, he can't discuss these areas with you.

At the same time, you need to *listen* to the doctor's evaluation of your present look. You may find yourself asking for the "moon."

An open dialogue is the most important start.

Be honest with yourself and be realistic about yourself.

Another guest at The Hidden Garden told me how she made her final decision. She went to three well-qualified doctors for a consultation. At forty-two she had a tired look. She wanted a picker-upper after her divorce. Doctor #1 recommended doing nothing just yet, "too young." He looked at her age, not at her. Doctor #2 recommended a cheek implant. Doctor #3 recommended a facelift. She knew she needed something, so Doctor #1 was definitely out of the picture. Doctor #3 was definitely wrong. "A facelift, at 42, forget it. I'm too young" ... Doctor #2 was her choice and seemed to her like the perfect solution. Her cheek implants helped, but, she still needs a facelift. She did not want to hear the real truth.

The Big Five-O used to be the age to have facelifts but not any longer. Men and women in their 40's outnumber any other age group. They are better candidates for surgery. They are healthier, heal better, have less trauma to the body, and it's easier to add another "nip and tuck" later. It is not a stigma to have a facelift at 44, 43, even 42 or 40.

A charming lady stayed at The Hidden Garden for six nights. She had a facelift. The day before her surgery she stopped by to leave her small suitcase. She "Be-bopped" up the stairs and "Be-bopped" down the stairs. When I picked her up from recovery, she looked fabulous. As night fell she asked to speak privately to our nurse and confided in her that she was frightened and that the nurse should know that the age she told her doctor, 68, was not true. She really was 78. She wanted the nurse to be alerted, just in case she developed any problems.

Nola's Note: She was on the Olympic Swim Team in the 30's and swam every day of her life!

Problems that occur with plastic surgery patients often occur when one is so obsessed by the desire for the change that they do not tell the doctor the whole truth. Perhaps they are afraid the doctor will not do the surgery.

Heavy drinkers often have nutritional deficiencies and can have liver problems hampering the body's ability to clot the blood.

Smokers are more likely to develop chest infections. Smoke contains carbon monoxide which is highly toxic to hemoglobin depriving it of oxygen. Less oxygen means slower healing time. It can cause high blood pressure which can mean more bleeding and bruising. Smoking is especially dangerous for a facelift.

AIDS is an extreme case. Some doctors will do plastic surgery on AIDS or HIV positive people. Most doctors don't.

There are doctors who will do surgery on anyone perhaps for the challenge, perhaps they get emotionally involved or perhaps for the price! A qualified doctor will require blood tests and EKGs ten days before surgery. If you are anemic or have an infection, a qualified doctor will postpone the surgery date.

It is most important for you to tell the Doctor:

1. If you are pregnant.

2. If you even think you might be pregnant.

3. If you are allergic to certain medications or foods.

4. If you have special medications you take daily.

5. If you have had plastic surgery done before, even years ago.

6. If you have high blood pressure. If you have low blood pressure.

7. If you have any medical problem or allergy.

8. If you have had any reaction to anesthesia before.

9. If you have bladder or urination difficulties.

10. If you are taking recreational drugs (cocaine, marijuana, etc.).

11. If you are under psychotherapy.

12. If you smoke. Tell the doctor how long and how many cigarettes per day.*

13. If you drink alcohol. And, how much.*

14. If you wear a wig.

15. Your real age!

*If you are a "Smoker," or heavy drinker, it is very important that both the surgeon and the anesthesiologist know this.

Once, again, an honest dialogue between you and your doctor including both physical and psychological reasons for the surgery should be discussed. The doctor must understand your expectations *and* your emotional problems to be able to realistically inform you of the results. Judy Didcoct, a favorite nurse at The Hidden Garden, reminds us, "Plastic surgery may be 'fun surgery,' but it is still surgery and should not be taken lightly."

Doctors talk of "results." You are going to have a wonderful "result." Does it mean:

1. You will look naturally younger, refreshed and uplifted. (Like Ivana Trump).

2. You will obviously look ten years younger? (Like Liz Taylor)

3. You will look "changed." (Like Michael Jackson)

Each doctor has his own idea of what "result" he wants. Does your idea of "result" match his?

A guest complained that she had been given ear lobes after her facelift. She had tiny ears that she loved and no creation of ear lobes was ever discussed. Her doctor had decided in surgery that she would look so much better with "ear lobes." She loved her new face but was very unhappy about her new ears.

ASK and **LISTEN**, and **ASK** again!

*It is just as important for the doctor to know what you
like about yourself as what you want to change.*

Looking Good: Count The Ways

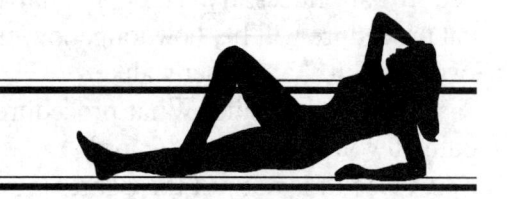

Although cosmetic surgery of the "aging face" has been around since the turn of the Century, surgical procedures have been fantastically improved over the past decade. Madame Dr. A. Noel was born in Lyon, France in 1878. A graduate from the Faculty of Medicine of Paris, she was one of the first women to practice cosmetic surgery exclusively, including the correction of baggy eyelids, double chins, scars and tattoos. In her book, *La Chirurgie Esthetique*, published in 1926, she wrote:

"Six case histories were presented in detail, five women and one man, all of whom had various procedures performed on their aging faces that were successful in helping them obtain employment and giving them remarkable self-confidence. The people were charmingly described as 'very refined,' 'of unquestionable taste,' 'a ruined high-class woman,' 'abandoned and ruined by her husband,' and 'from the plebeian class.' Initially, she operated only on desperate cases but later on others, motivated by the 'love of finery and beauty.'

In describing the age at which people should seek surgery, she stated, 'I am forced to send every candidate to his or her mirror.' It is also clear that her procedures needed to be redone frequently, as often as yearly. But in defense she emphasized that many parts of the body need frequent maintenance. Many of her patients apparently underwent several staged procedures a few days to weeks apart. She went to lengths to indicate that with her operations the scars were invisible and that with a slight change in hair style or a new hat the healing incisions could be camouflaged. One Serbian woman physician had her surgery at six o'clock in the evening, wearing her evening dress, because she was having dinner at the embassy at eight.

The comforting, supportive, and understanding atmosphere that Noel provided for her patients is as important now as it was 60 years ago. Although our surgical approach to the aging face has changed dramatically, the motivation of our patients and the emotional rewards to the patients and surgeons have not changed."[4]

Cosmetic surgery has become more and more popular among people from all walks of life and is no longer limited to the rich and famous. People just want to look better.

You and the consulting surgeon can discuss more accurately the changes in your face and body and what results to expect if you understand the cosmetic procedures that are involved in the correction of the "aging face." A full facelift is made up of several procedures. There are anterior facelifts, there are forehead lifts, necklifts, browlifts, chemical peels, etc. Often several surgical procedures are necessary. The combination of facial work will depend on how extensive your surgical procedure will be, how long, how expensive, and how much recuperation will be necessary. No two "facelifts" are exactly alike.

What is a facelift? What procedure or combination of procedures do you need? Will a facelift cure all your problems of aging?

A facelift is not just the tightening of skin; it is much more involved. Most facelift cosmetic surgery candidates aren't really interested in the actual technical surgical procedure. You can skip this part if you want. One guest came to The Hidden Garden with her camera. She had had the nurse in surgery take pictures as the doctor performed. Another guest had her surgery video taped. This is very unusual.

Most guests do not want to know the exact cutting details. But just in case you do...

Rhytidectomy/Facelift:

The facial skin loses its elasticity and causes drooping and lines. Pronounced folds appear that run from the side of the nose to the edges of the mouth. The cheekbones lose definition. The jawline has jowls. The earlobes lengthen. Folds of skin appear on the neck, often referred to as the "Turkey" neck, are the number one sign of aging. Sometimes the neck or platysma muscle is greatly accentuated like two heavy cords. Treatment of these conditions is usually referred to as a "facelift."

The incision for the facelift begins in the hair at the temple and extends to a point in the hair above the ear. From that point the incision continues downward following the natural line in front of and immediately within the ear folds. The incision continues down in this narrow shallow groove before it goes behind the earlobe into the hair of the scalp. Actually quite inconspicuous. This allows for minimal scarring and allows one to wear her hair "up". (Note: Men usually have their incisions in front of the ear, the incision is hidden at the facial point where the beard ends and the ear begins.) The design of these incisions varies from patient to patient according to the surgeon. No two facelifts are alike.

Surgical techniques differ but basically the skin is elevated and stretched, facial muscles are tightened, and excess fat removed. Care must be taken not to injure the facial nerve. When completed, the skin is pulled upward and backward with tacking sutures to hold incisions together.

An excellent result usually occurs when both a facelift and a peel procedure are combined. Collagen or fat injections may be used to contour the new look.

Look good: Seven to fourteen days

Final shape: Four to six months

Nola's Note: A facelift will soften major facial expression lines. A peel may be necessary to soften and remove wrinkles often found on the upper lip and under the eyes.

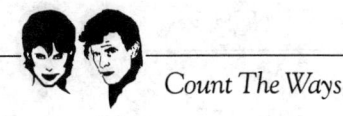

Anterior or Mini-facelift:

As the facial skin loses its elasticity, facial gestures accentuate the prominence of the "nasolabial" folds, "smile lines". Sometimes the downward displacement of tissues from the cheek produces jowls and a square-looking face.

In a mini-lift, usually no neck work is involved, but incisions around the ears are made.

Look good: seven to ten days

Final shape: four weeks

Coronoplasty (Forehead or Browlift):

Signs of aging are evident not only in the general skin texture but forehead lines have deepened and are more evident. Especially unattractive and distressing are the vertical frown lines between the eyebrows. Usually, eyebrows have fallen. The so-called "crow's feet," lines running outward from the eyelid become especially apparent with smiling.

An incision is made either just at the hairline or behind the hairline, depending on exactly where the individual hairline is and the hairstyle worn.

Look good: two weeks

Final shape: eight to twelve weeks

Blepharoplasty (Eyelid Surgery):

Sad, tired eyes can make a face look old before any other signs of aging. The excess skin creating droopiness in the upper lids and the accumulation of fat in the lower lids cause the "baggy" eye look. Because this tendency is inherited, it can appear in one's late twenties or early thirties. Other causes can be excessive sun, excessive alcohol and smoking.

The incision for the upper eyelid is made in the normal eyelid crease and therefore hardly seen. The lower eyelid incision is made at the very edge of the lid, at the base of the eyelashes. In some cases, the incision is made inside the lower eyelid and no exterior stitches are used.

Look good: five to ten days

Final shape: four to six weeks

Rhinoplasty (Nose Surgery):

Probably the most popular surgery with regards to cosmetic procedures is nose surgery. A natural but attractive nose is in high demand. No longer do patients want that short, upturned nose, the rage of the fifties, but a more natural nose, a nose that belongs with the face. All work is done inside the nose: bumps sanded and cartilage removed or relocated to re-shape the nose. At times cartilage from one's ear can be used to create a new shaped nose.

Packing inside the nose is sometimes required for one to five days, "Instead of packing, some surgeons use 'Doyle splints.' These silastic splints allow the patient to breathe immediately following surgery and usually, their removal is painless."[5] The sutures inside the nose are dissolvable.

Look good: three weeks

Final shape: twelve months

Nola's Note: As we age, the tip of the nose droops, the nasal bridge becomes prominent. A straight nose may develop a bump.

Mentoplasty (Chin Implant):

A common complaint is a recessed or underdeveloped chin. Ideally, the chin should project to a point immediately below the lower lip. An implant can be inserted to augment one's existing chin. Usually the sutures are inside the mouth under the lower lip, or under the chin.

Look good: ten days to two weeks

Final look: three to six months

Malarplasty (Cheek Implant):

Cheek implants can improve facial contour. Our society places a beauty star on high cheek bones. Implants can be placed either through an incision in the mouth or below the eyelashes of the lower lids or inside the lower lid. The implants are sutured in place and an occasional external stitch is used temporarily. If a facelift is also being considered, it can be done along with this procedure.

Look good: three weeks

Final look: three to four months

Mastopexy (Breast Lift):

A breast lift can improve loose, sagging breasts that have lost volume and elasticity after child bearing. The internal breast tissue is reduced and reshaped and the nipple is relocated. The breast may be reduced (reduction mammoplasty) or augmented at this time. This procedure usually involves some scarring.

Breast Augmentation/Augmentation Mammoplasty:

Marked sagging of the breasts, small or underdeveloped breasts or breasts that have decreased in size or atrophied after child-bearing are the most common reasons for an augmentation. You should discuss size and contour with your surgeon. Augmentation may also be considered to achieve asymmetry resulting from post-mastectomy reconstruction.

Three techniques are usually considered:

- An incision made under the breast;
- An incision made around the dark pink skin that surrounds the nipple;
- An incision made in the armpit.

The implant may then be placed either in a pocket directly under the breast tissue or under the chest muscle. You and your surgeon will make the best decision for your anatomy.

The saline breast implants placed *under the chest muscle* seem to be very satisfactory. When the implant is not oversized, but appropriate to the natural cup size, an excellent and happy result can be seen and enjoyed. The chest muscle allows for the most natural look and feel with little, if any, "swishing." Women feel safe and comfortable with this procedure. The final look is excellent.

Look good: ten to fourteen days

Final look: five to six months

Breast Reduction/Reduction Mammoplasty:

This breast reduction procedure is both cosmetic and functional. Women not only look better, feel less self-conscious, but chronic discomfort from neck, shoulder and back pain can be relieved.

There are a number of techniques used to remove excess tissue from large breasts to create a smaller, firmer shape. The surgeon may use a combination of these techniques. But the typical procedure would involve an incision circling the areola of the nipple and going down to the crease under the breast. Excessive tissue, fat and skin are removed. The nipple is often repositioned higher on the new breast. When skillfully performed, the resulting scars can be almost totally unnoticeable.

Look good: ten to fourteen days

Final look: five to six months

Abdominoplasty (Tummy Tuck):

Frequently, diet and exercise alone cannot get rid of the excess skin, fat and stretched-out abdominal muscles often due to multiple pregnancies or excessive weight loss. Patients who maintain a steady weight but have weak abdominal muscles, excess skin and fat are the best candidates.

The surgeon's procedure is to remove excess abdominal skin and tighten the underlying muscle. The umbilicus (belly button!) is freed from the surrounding skin and is reinstated, creating a new navel.

Look good: twelve to fourteen days

Final look: two to three months

Nola's Note: *This is not a substitute for weight reduction.*

Suction-Assisted Lipectomy/Liposuction:

Good candidates are of normal weight with elastic skin but have localized collections of excessive fat, protruding abdomen, large hips and thighs. Facial contouring areas under the chin or cheeks, as well as removal of fat on arms, calves, knees and above the waist, "love handles," are all successfully performed by this procedure.

A tiny incision is made through the skin in the selected area. A tubular instrument with a suction unit attached is passed through the incision into the area under the skin. The surgeon manipulates the instrument while suctioning off the fat. Liposuction from several areas of the body seems safe up to 1500 ccs of fat and fluid. After that, a blood transfusion may be necessary. It is very important that when considering this procedure to go to a Board Certified Surgeon who is very skilled with liposuction and who understands blood and fluid loss and replacement and can handle potential complications. The magic number here is the removal of 1500 ccs. If the doctor feels he will come close to that amount, you should give your blood in advance to be saved and replaced. At least one pint is needed. If the surgeon feels he may go over that magic number, give two pints of your blood to be on hold for your safety. There is no need to use someone else's blood when you can prepare yourself for this possibility. The American Blood Institute will gladly take your blood and give it back to you for your surgery.

"The patient's skin must be somewhat elastic so that after the fat is removed, the skin is able to recontour to the new shape. People who have undergone very large fluctuations in their body weight are often poor candidates for liposuction. The quality of the skin in these patients is very poor, lacking the necessary elasticity. In these patients, it is usually necessary to remove the loose skin as well as the excess fat.... Generally, liposuction will not improve cellulite."

"*Will the fat come back?* Liposuction removes fat cells that, once removed, will not come back, since it is thought that no new fat cells are produced after puberty. Since it is not desirable to re move *all* fat from an area, there *are* fat cells remaining and these cells *can* get larger if a significant amount of weight is gained. However, the previous "bulges" will not return."

"A snug elastic garment will be placed over the suctioned areas after the surgery is completed. This garment will help control swelling and bleeding, and will help the skin mold to the new contour. Generally, these garments are worn continuously for 2-3 weeks and then worn only during the day for an additional 2-3 weeks. Bicycle shorts or support panty hose may be worn in place of the surgical garment after the first 2-3 weeks."

"Immediately after surgery the patient may notice very little change because swelling will mask the improvement. There will also be some bruising and numbness in the areas suctioned, since the small nerves leading to the skin are interrupted and need to be reconnected after surgery.... Bruising, if present, can persist for a week or more. Swelling, however, may persist longer. The final result may not be evident for several months, but the vast majority of swelling is gone in a matter of weeks."

If waviness or contour problems occur, these problems can be corrected easily with a minor revision under local anesthesia. Excess fat can be suctioned if present. If a depression in the skin has occurred, fat can be injected into the area to correct the problem.[6]

To encourage skin shrinkage a long-legged girdle must be worn for one to two months.

Look good: two to three weeks

Final look: three to four months

Nola's Note: *Liposuction is not a substitute for weight reduction that can be attained through diet and exercise. It is not a cure for obesity.*

Buttock Lift:

Saggy or flabby buttocks can be surgically improved. This procedure is performed under the buttock. An incision is made, excessive fat and skin is removed, the muscle tightened and reinforced.

Look good: two to three weeks

Final look: one to five months

Chemosurgery/Peels:

A facelift cannot eliminate the fine vertical lines near the upper and lower lips and around the eyes. Crows-feet and fine lip lines from aging or effects of acne or other skin blemishes can be treated with a chemical solution to peel away the top layers of skin. During the healing process a new skin surface develops. Chemical peels often are an additional procedure with a facelift, the fine tuning a facelift needs. The peel takes four to five days to crust or dry out. The actual peeling or sloughing off of skin cells, will begin on or about the fifth day. New skin will appear, pink and very soft. The skin must be protected from the sun. Olive skin tones because of their deep pigmentation may not be good candidates, but ask a qualified and experienced surgeon. Careful consideration should be given to the deep Phenol peel procedure. It is painful and requires anesthesia. The Trichloracetic acid peel, often referred to as the "light" peel, is less serious and may be repeated if necessary. There are many different strengths of chemical peels available.

Dermabrasion:

This procedure is effective when one has scarring and deep pits from the results of severe acne or chicken pox and very deep aging lines or when one needs to remove pre-cancerous lesions. A highly sophisticated mechanical device sands smooth the areas concerned.

A lovely young lady, 34, came to The Hidden Garden for seven days. She had contracted "chicken pox" in her early thirties. She complained that her scars were as deep as a pencil's eraser. She was despondent. The deep, disfiguring pox scars not only destroyed her current relationships and her social life, but her career as well. After several consultations she selected a Board Certified Surgeon who carefully performed a full face dermabrasion. After a week, one could clearly see the incredible results of her new skin and the start of a new life.

This procedure may be performed with a chemical peel or facelift.

Look good: ten days

Final look: two to three weeks

Collagen:

Collagen Replacement Therapy is excellent for parts of the face that were not handled in surgery. Fine facial wrinkles and lines may be reduced with collagen injections. They are only necessary two to four times a year and are an excellent way to keep your new look.

Final look: one day

Fat Injections:

Taking fat from one part of the body and injecting it into another area has the advantage of a longer lasting effect than collagen. The body accepts its own fat easily.

Patients choose the donor site, usually the lower abdomen or hips. The most popular placement is in the facial folds, "the smile lines," the jawline and the lips. Where there is constant muscle action, the faster the displacement of the fat will occur. An average of three injections four to twelve months apart gives a satisfactory, lasting result. The leaner the patient, the less resorption, therefore requiring only one or two injections. The long term retention is 10-20% for each injection.

Final look: one week

> *"A woman's beauty is her most valuable asset. Every woman owes it to herself to look as good as she can and avail herself of every possible aid to increase her attractiveness...within the scope of Plastic Surgery, the beautiful are enabled to retain their beauty and the unattractive are made attractive."*[7]

The Hollywood Facelift

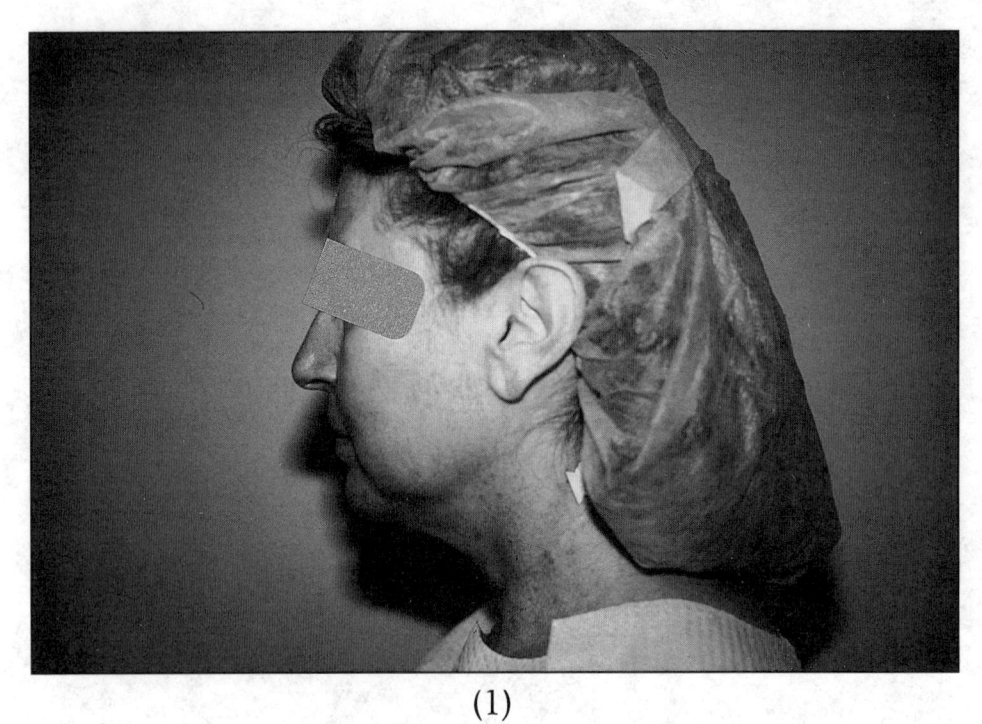

(1)
Facelift, neck and jowl defatting
Upper and lower eyes / Nasal reconstruction / Earlobe reduction
Before

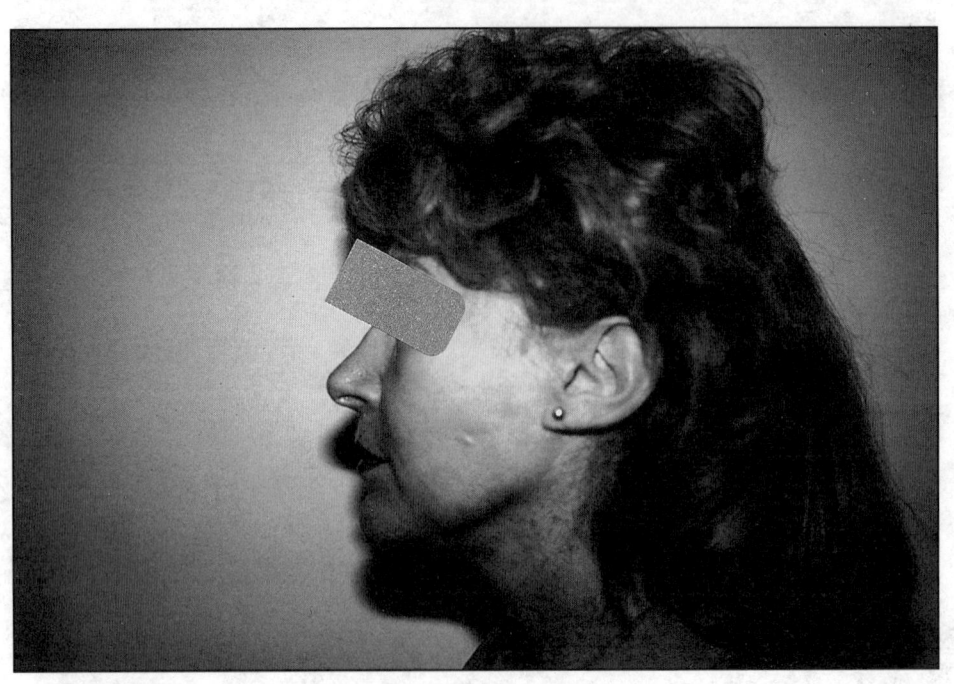

(2)
After
Photographs courtesy of Gary Tearston, M.D.

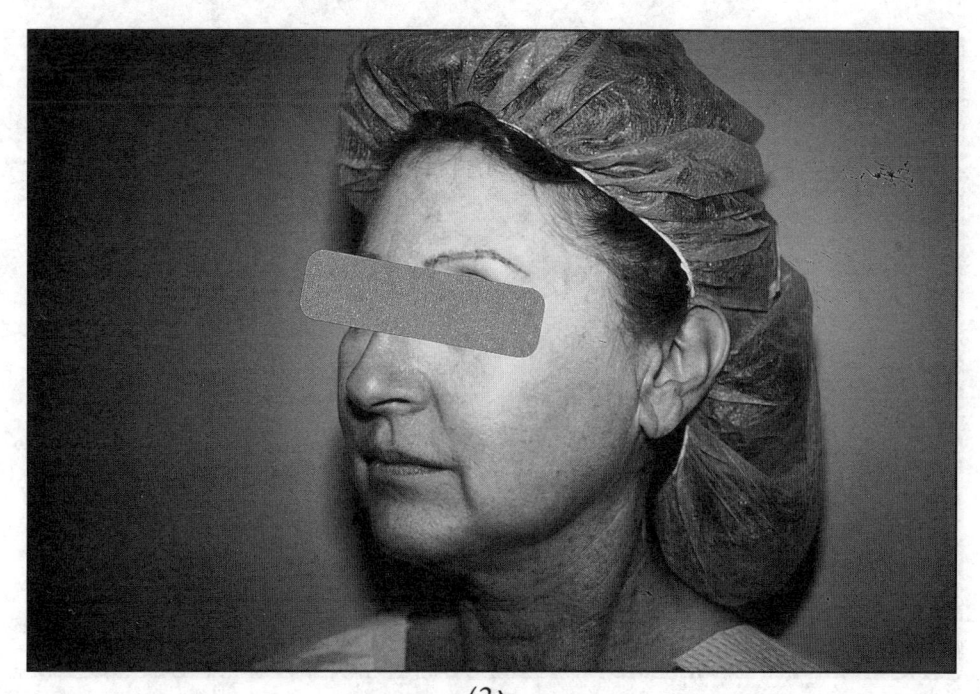

Looking Good: Count The Ways

(3)
Facelift, neck and jowl defatting
Upper and lower eyes / Nasal reconstruction / Earlobe reduction
Before

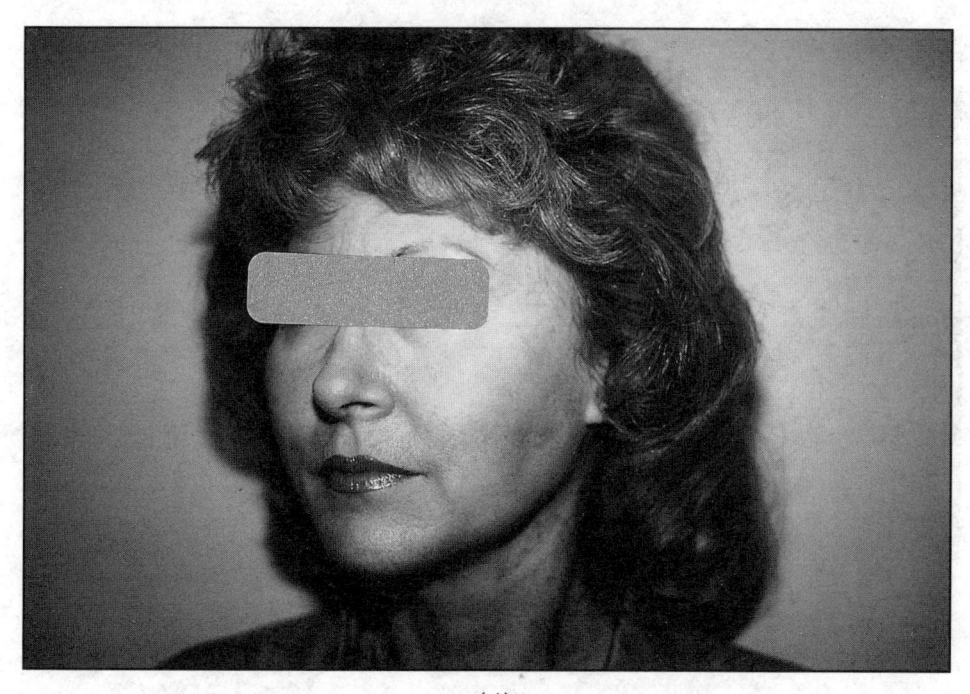

(4)
After

Photographs courtesy of Gary Tearston, M.D.

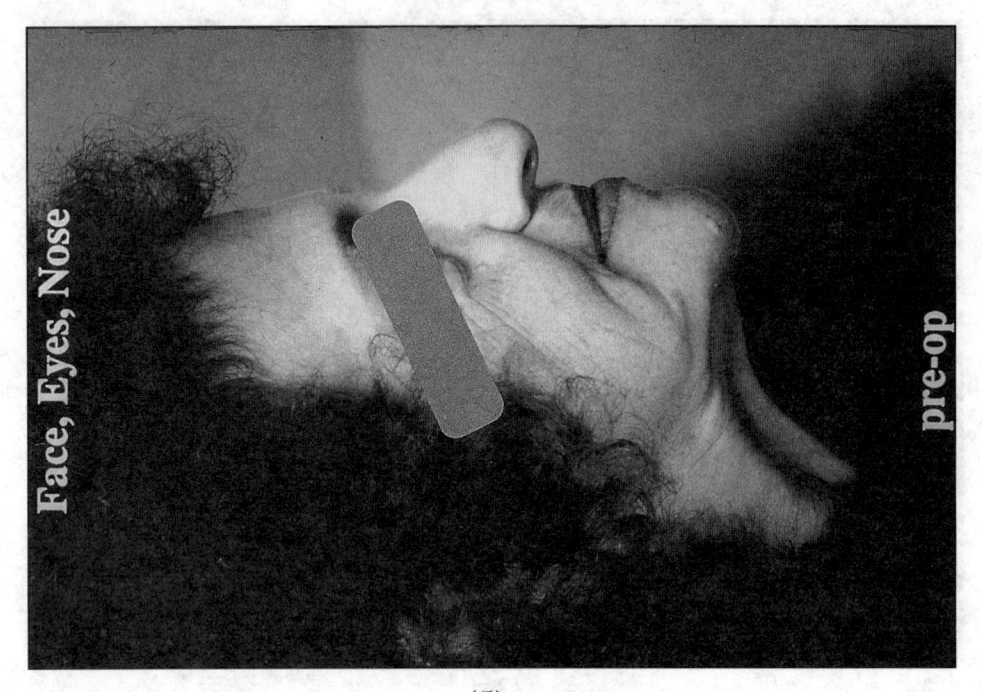

The Hollywood Facelift

(5)
Face, eyes and nose
Before

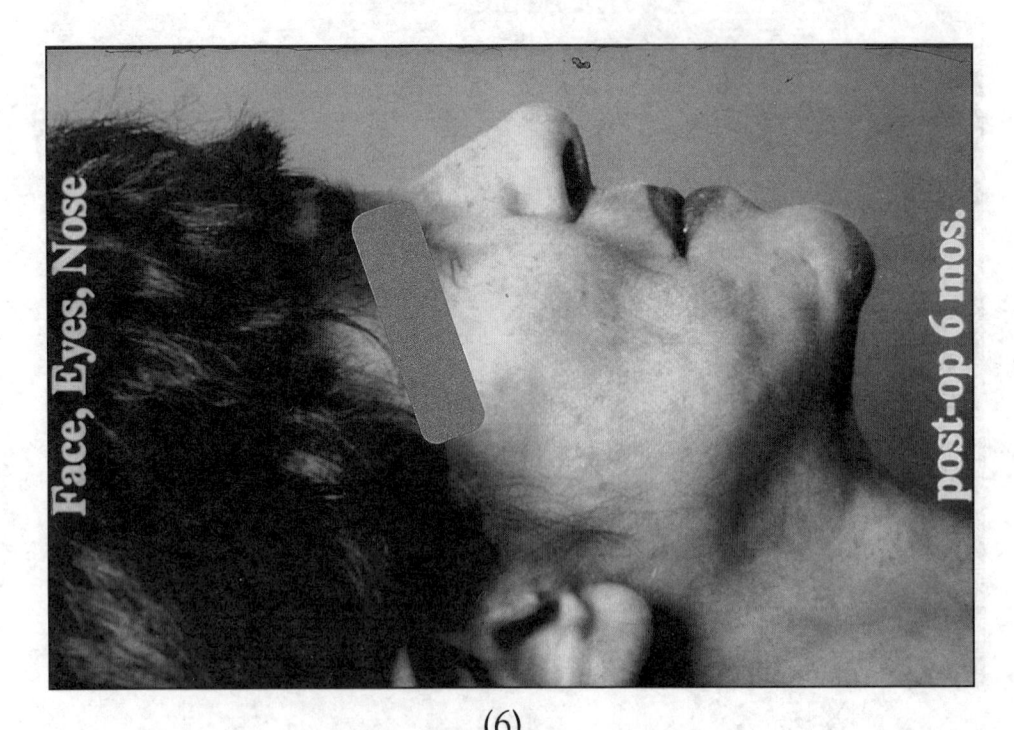

(6)
After

Photographs courtesy of Michael Churukian, M.D.

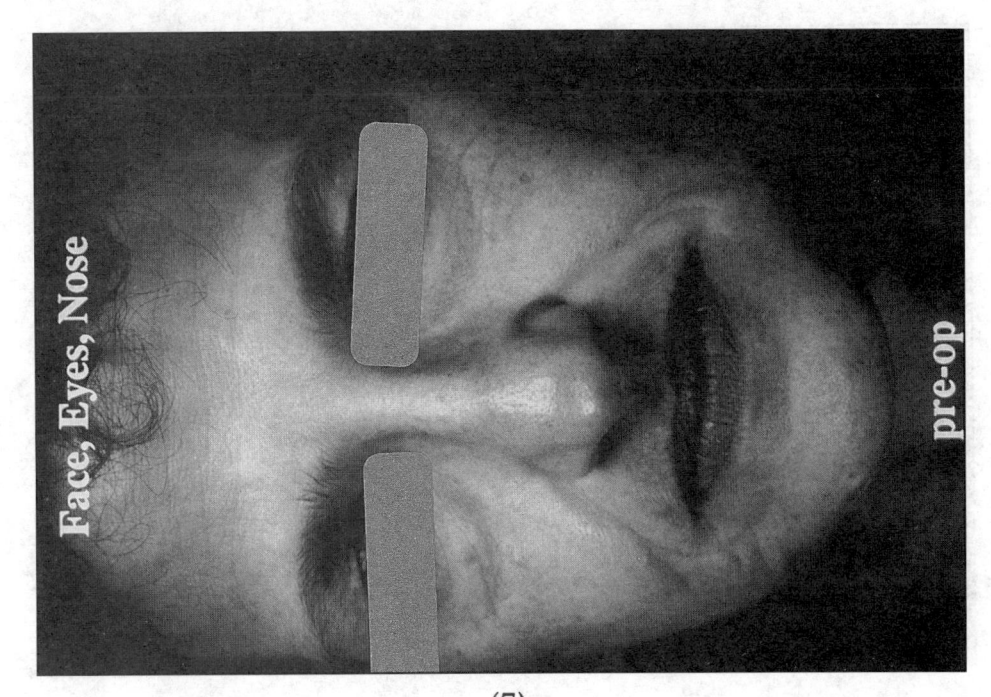

Looking Good: Count The Ways

(7)
Face, eyes, and nose
Before

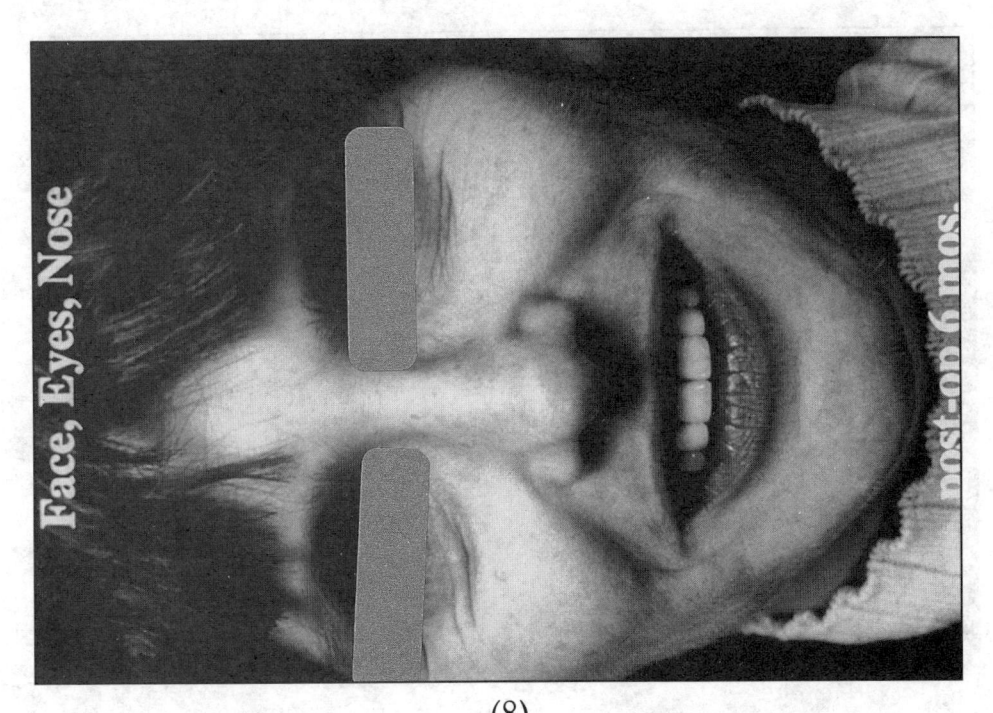

(8)
After

Photographs courtesy of Michael Churukian, M.D.

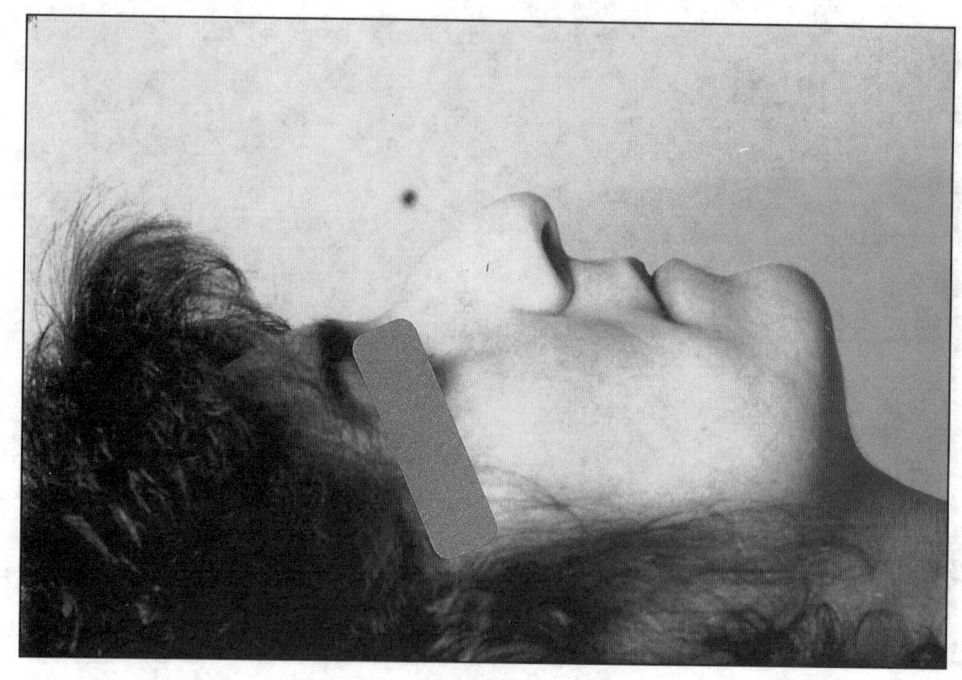

★ 38 ★

The Hollywood Facelift

(9)
Nasal reconstruction
Before

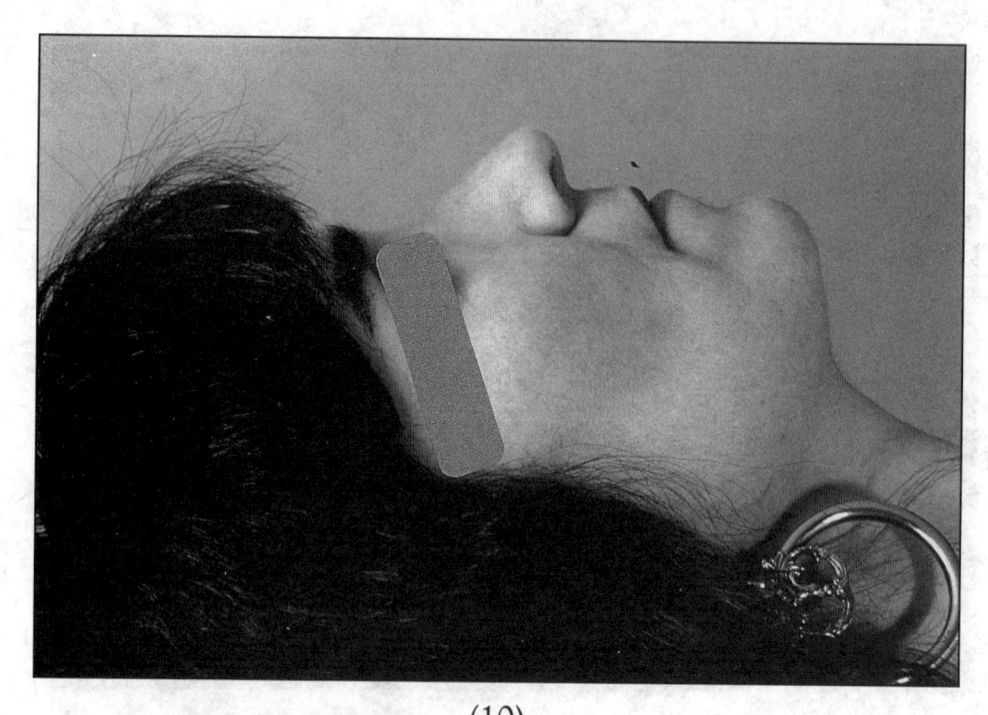

(10)
After

Photographs courtesy of Michael Churukian, M.D.

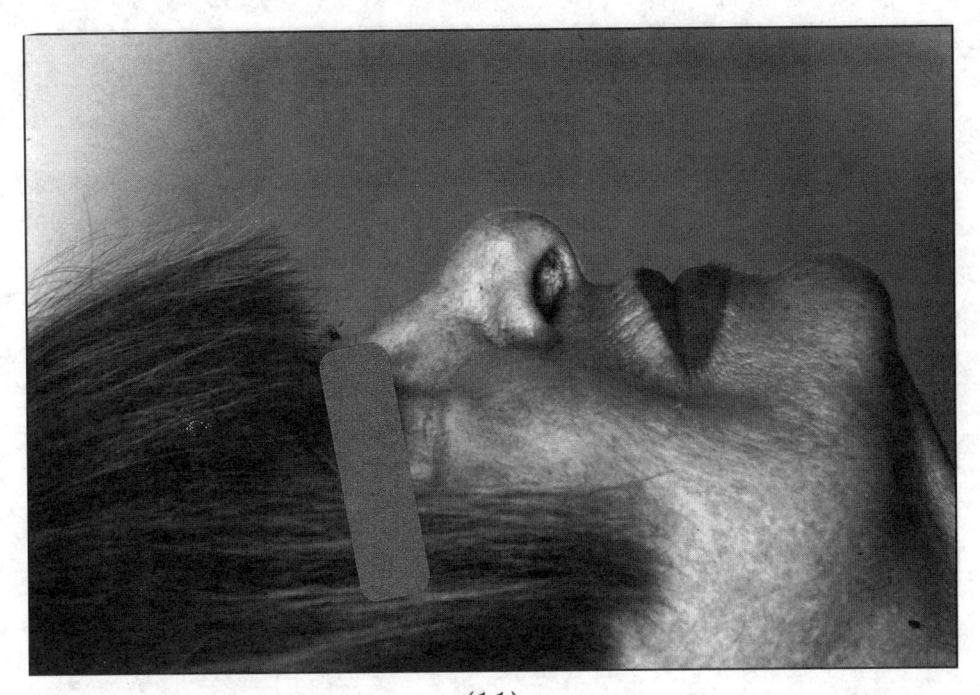

Looking Good: Count The Ways

(11)
Nose revision
Before

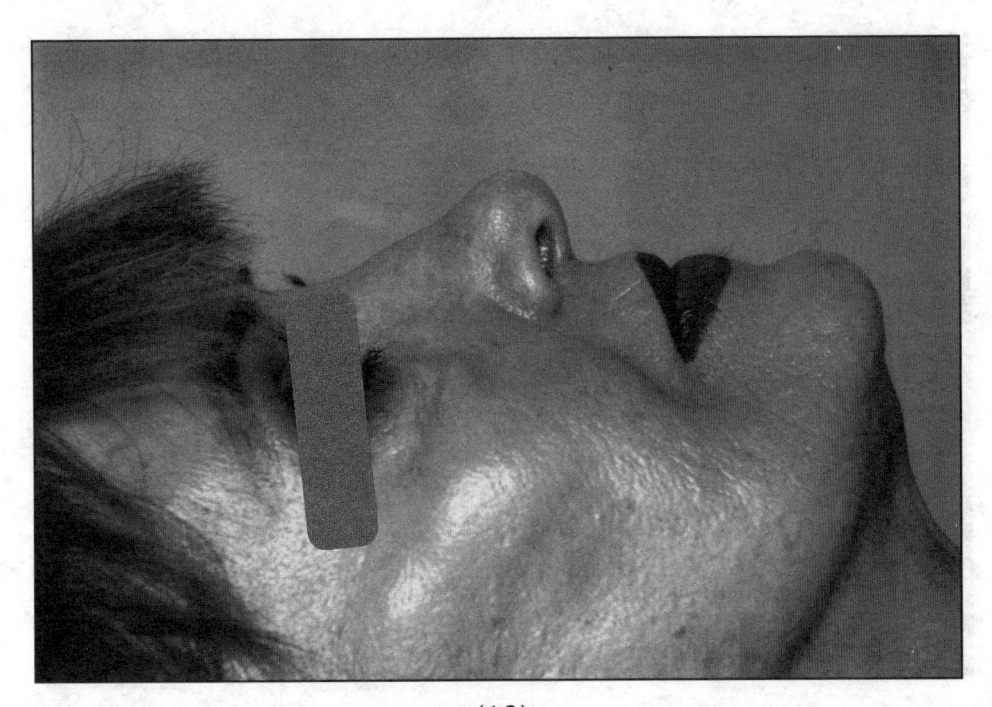

(12)
After

Photographs courtesy of Michael Churukian, M.D.

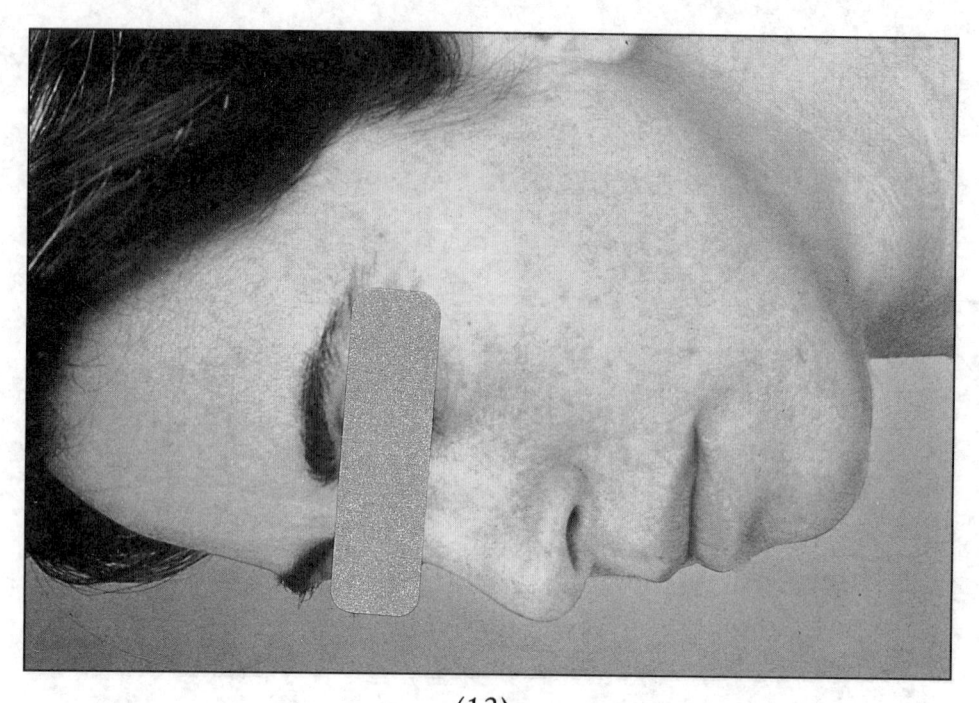

(13)
Nose, cheek and chin implants
Before

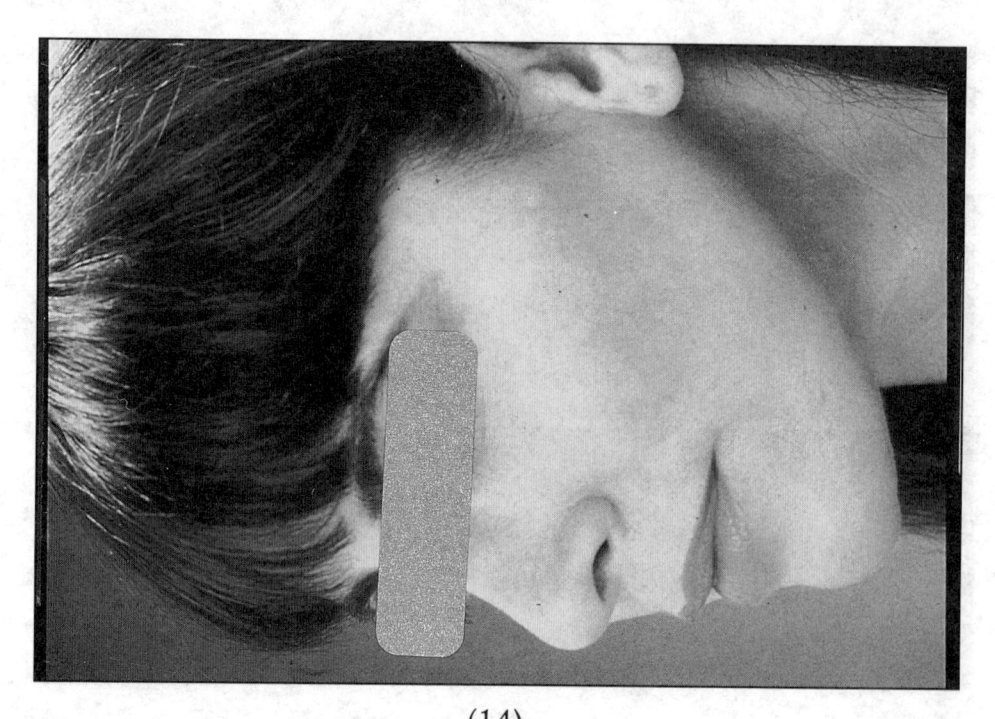

(14)
After

Photographs courtesy of John Williams, M.D.

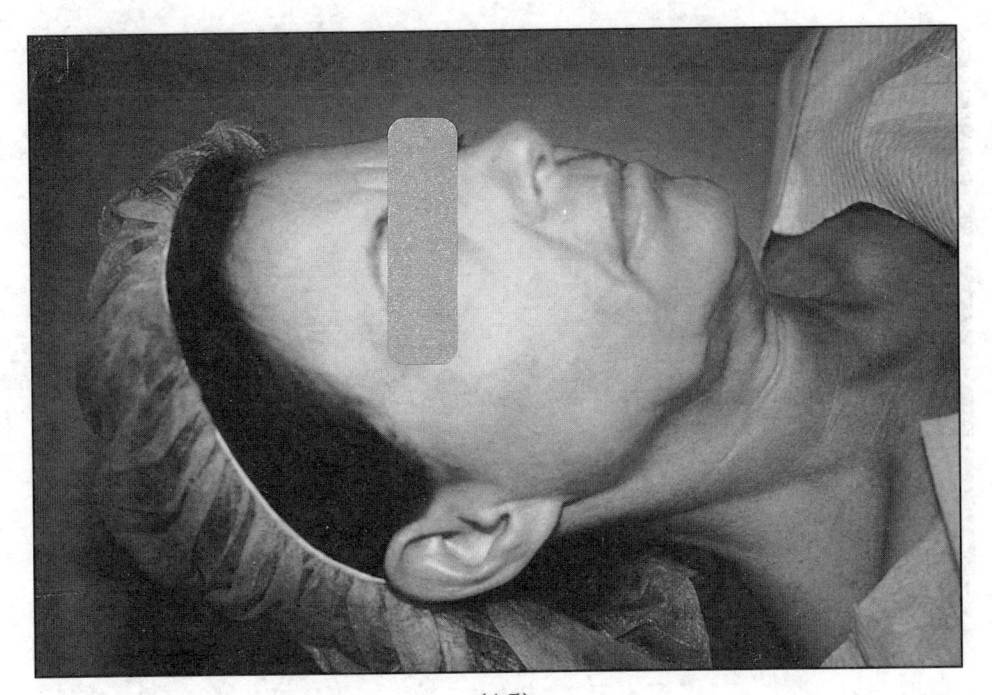

Looking Good: Count The Ways

(15)
Forehead lift, Facelift and upper and lower eyes
Before

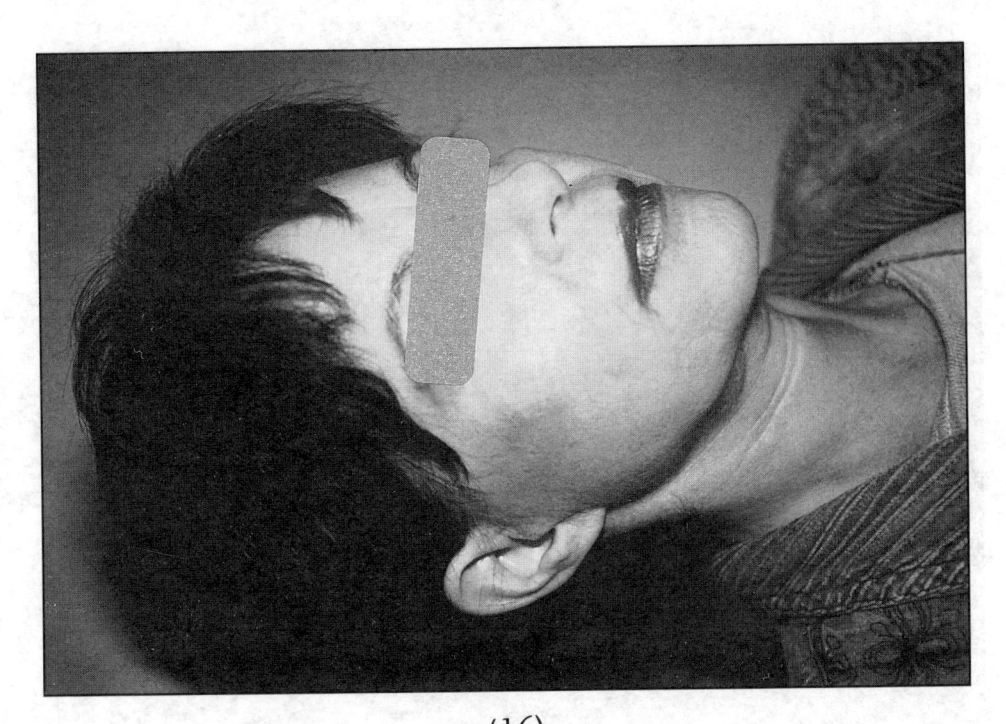

(16)
After

Photographs courtesy of Gary Tearston, M.D.

The Hollywood Facelift

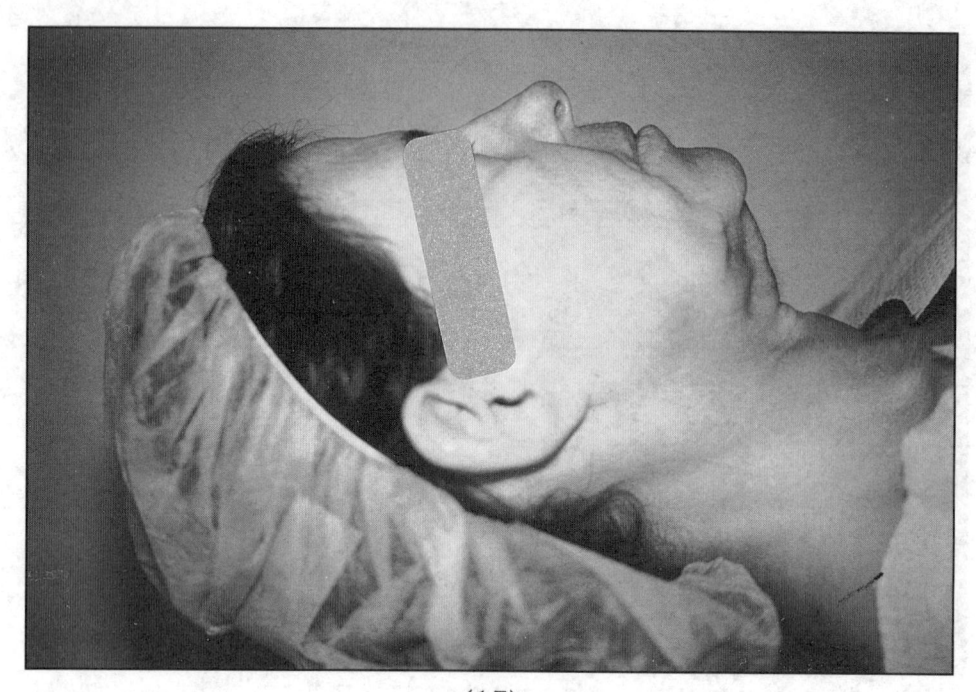

(17)
Forehead lift, Facelift and upper and lower eyes
Before

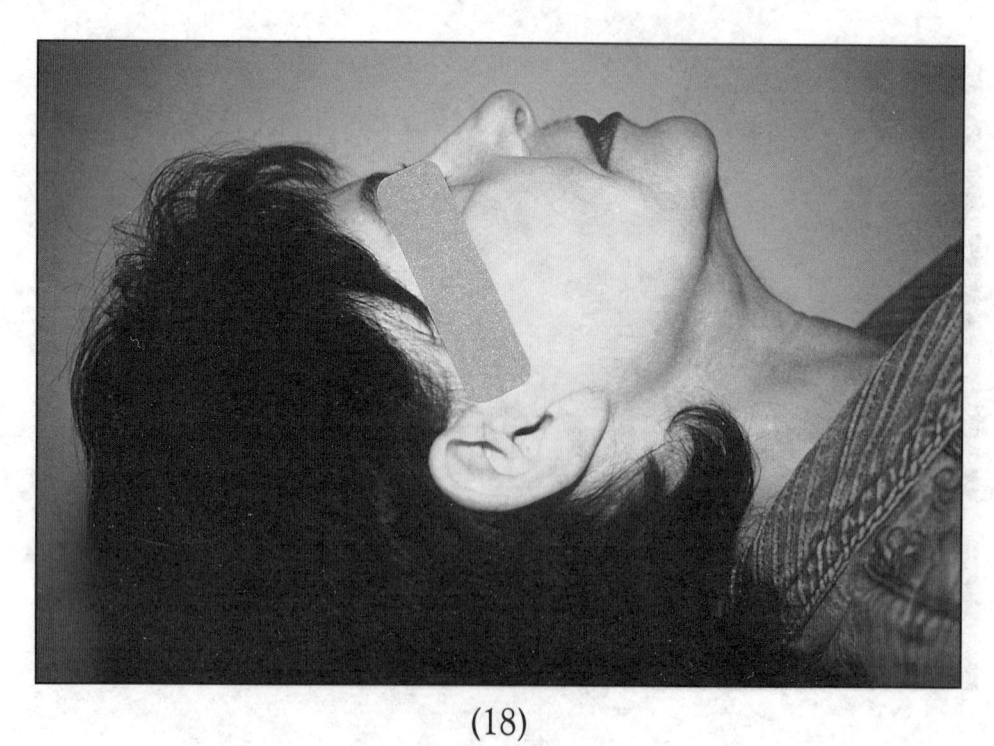

(18)
After

Photographs courtesy of Gary Tearston, M.D.

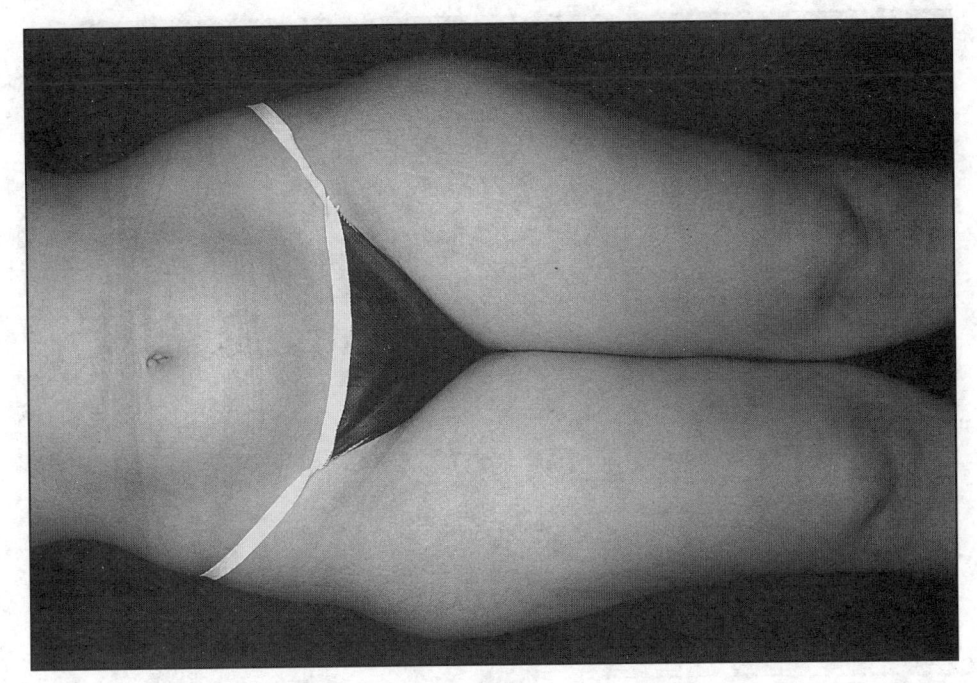

★ 43 ★

Looking Good: Count The Ways

(19)
Liposuction: Legs and abdomen
Before

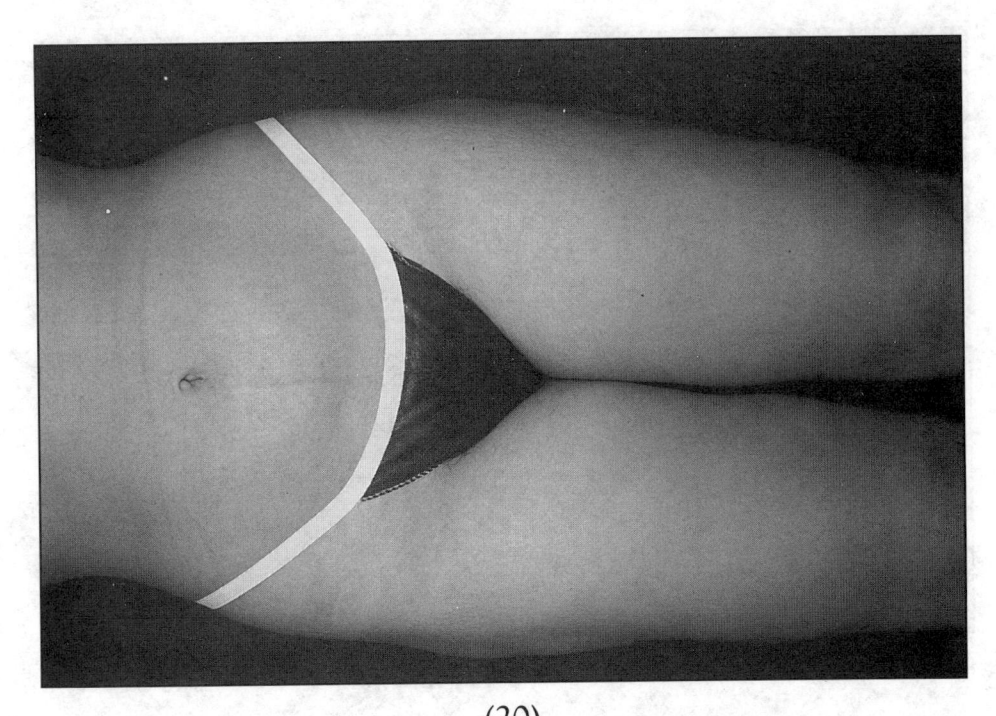

(20)
After

Photographs courtesy of Gary Tearston, M.D.

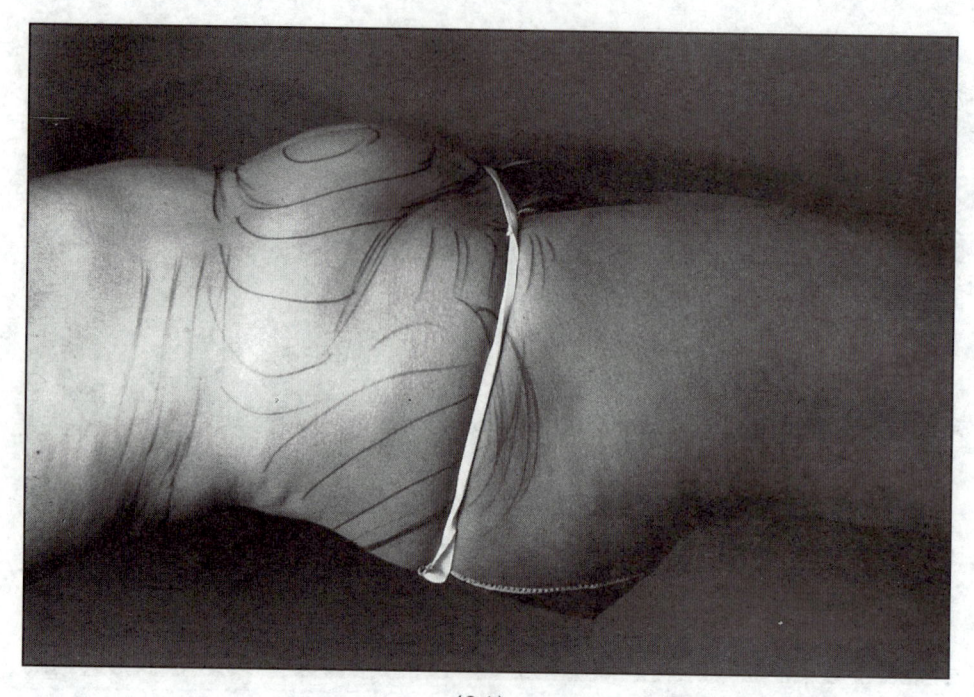

★ 44 ★

The Hollywood Facelift

(21)
Liposuction female: Legs, thighs and abdomen
Before

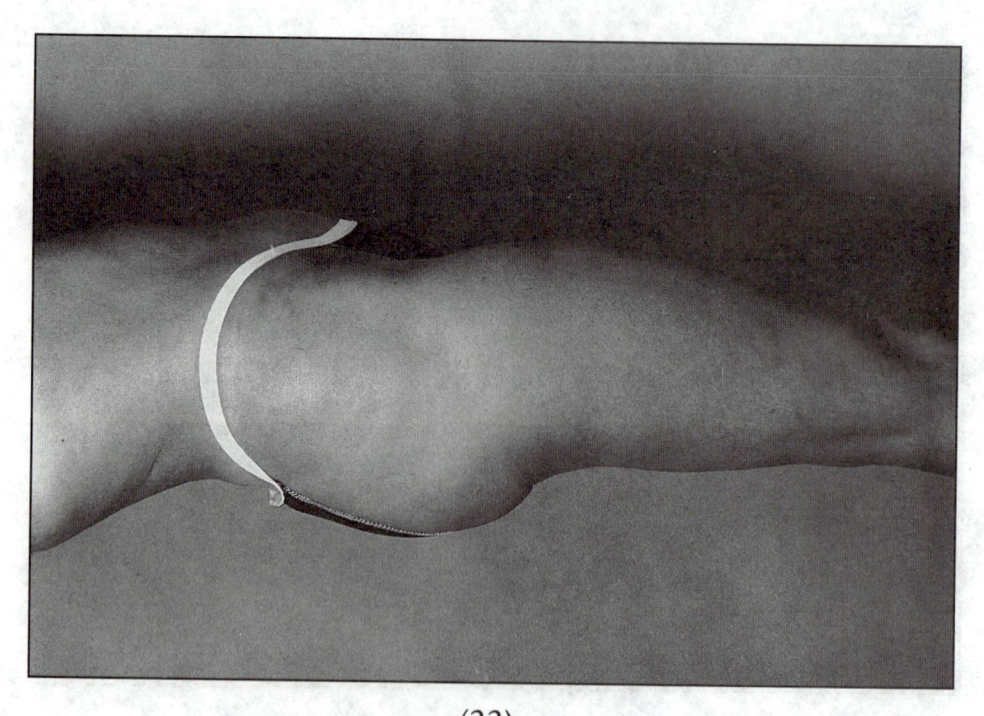

(22)
After

Photographs courtesy of Michael Churukian, M.D.

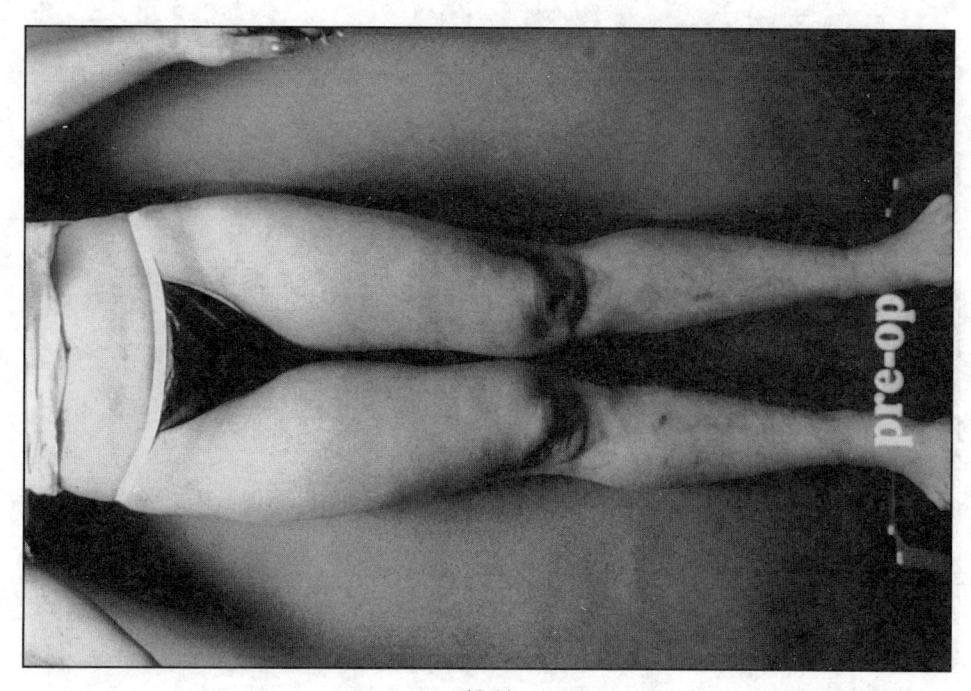

Looking Good: Count The Ways

(23)
Liposuction female: Ankles, calves, knees and thighs
Before

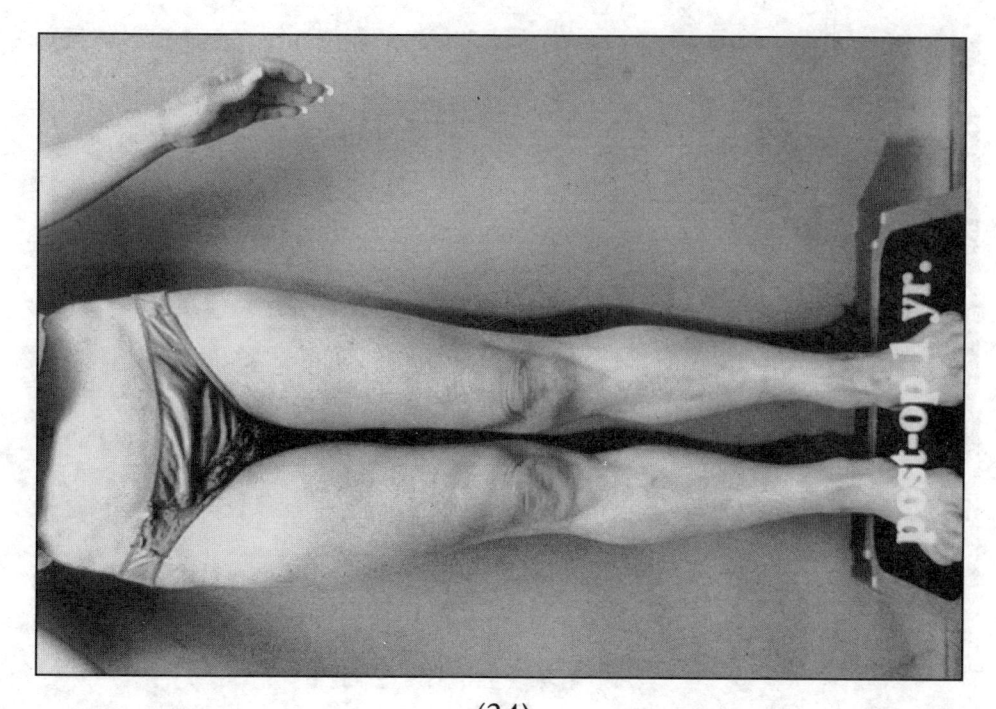

(24)
After

Photographs courtesy of Michael Churukian, M.D.

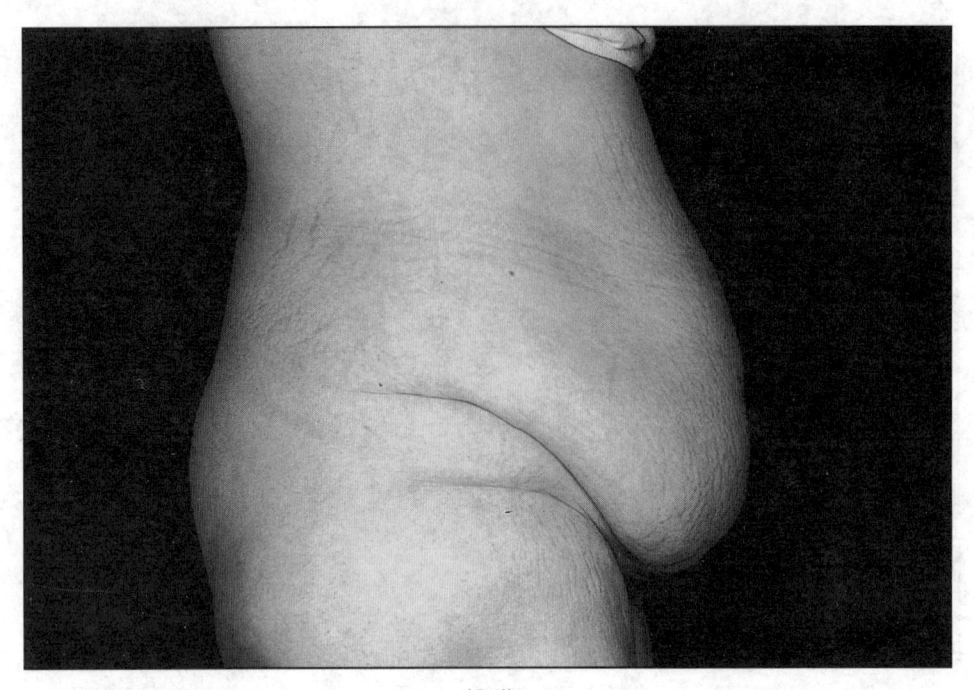

(25)
Tummy tuck
Before

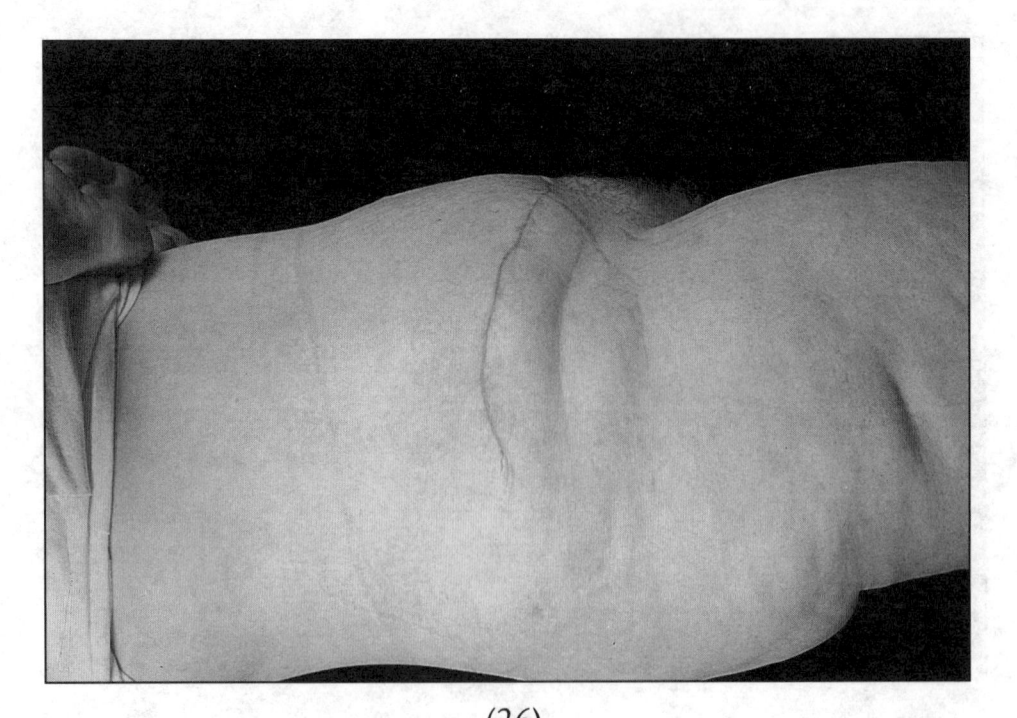

(26)
After

Photographs courtesy of Garth Fisher, M.D.

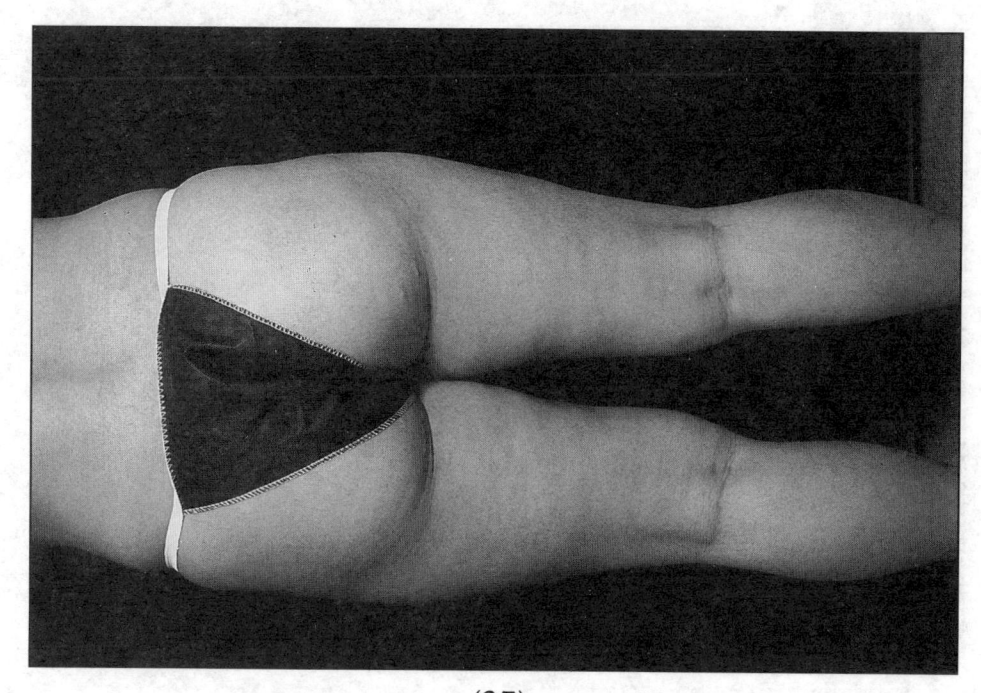

Looking Good: Count The Ways

(27)
Liposuction
Before

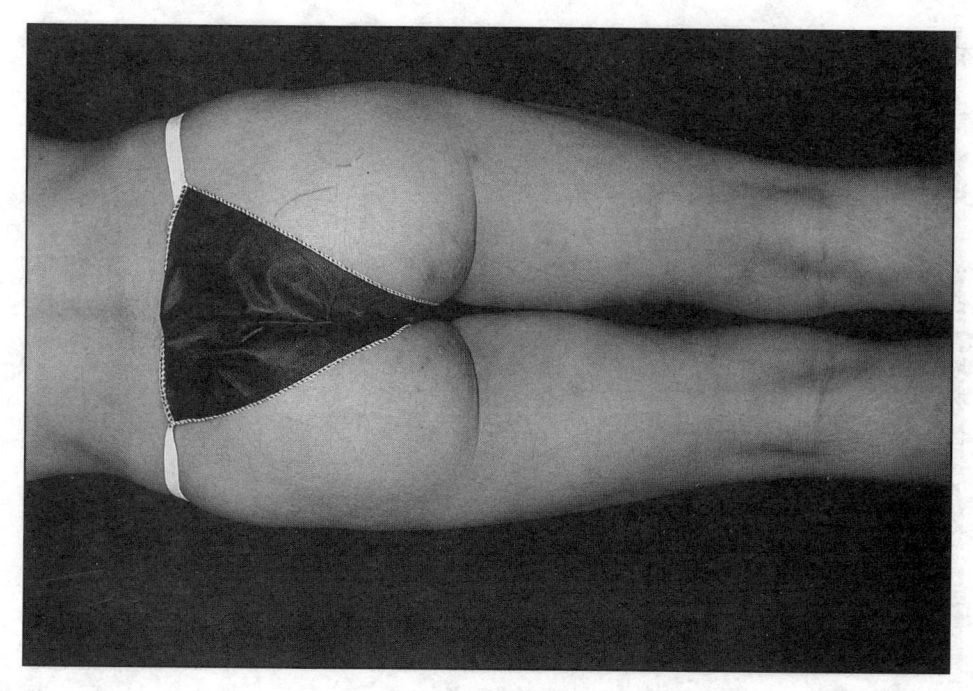

(28)
After

Photographs courtesy of Garth Fisher, M.D.

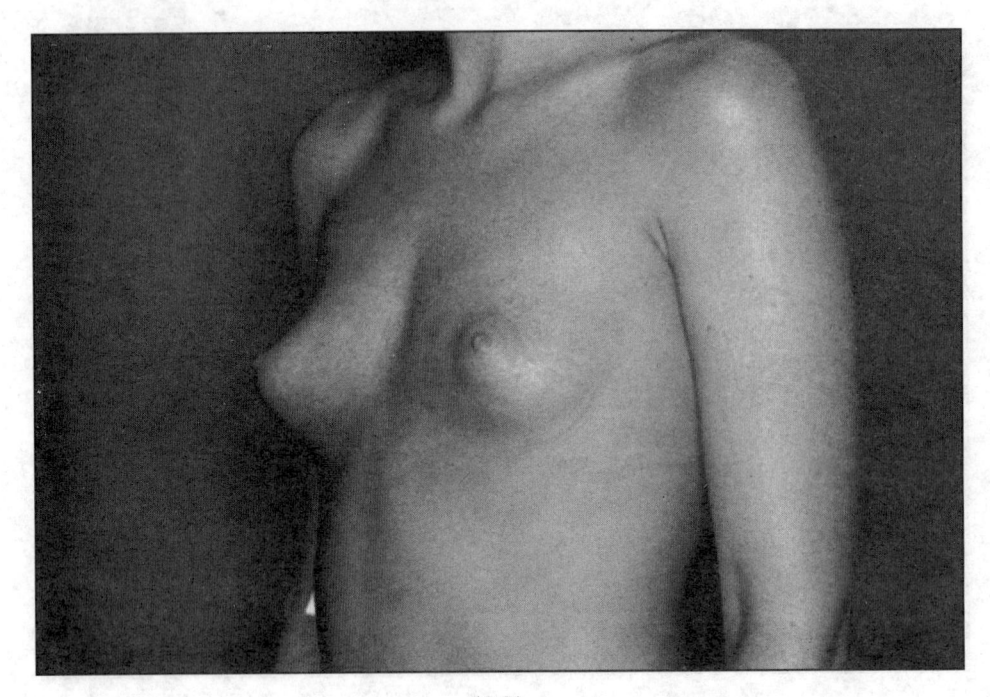

★ 48 ★

The Hollywood Facelift

(29)
Breast augmentation
Before

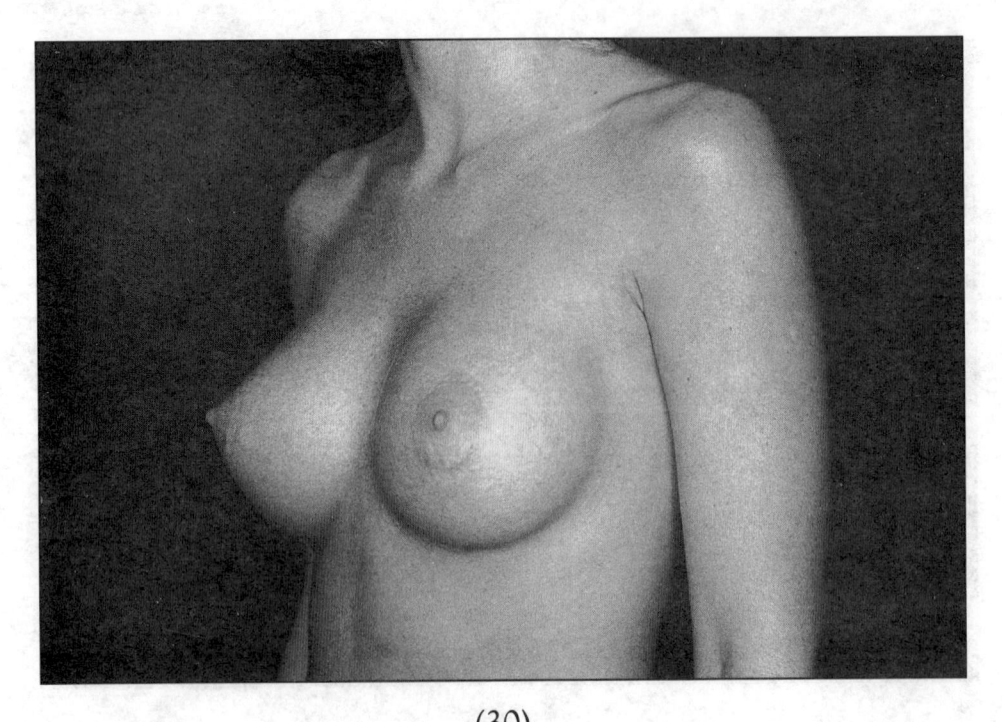

(30)
After

Photographs courtesy of Garth Fisher, M.D.

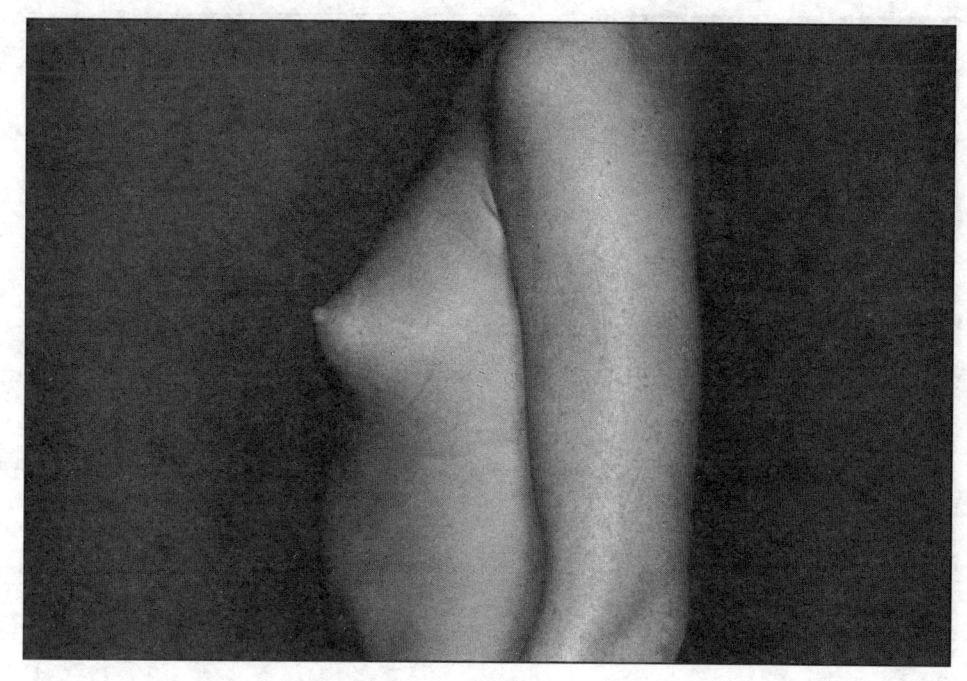

Looking Good: Count The Ways

★ 49 ★

(31)
Breast augmentation
Before

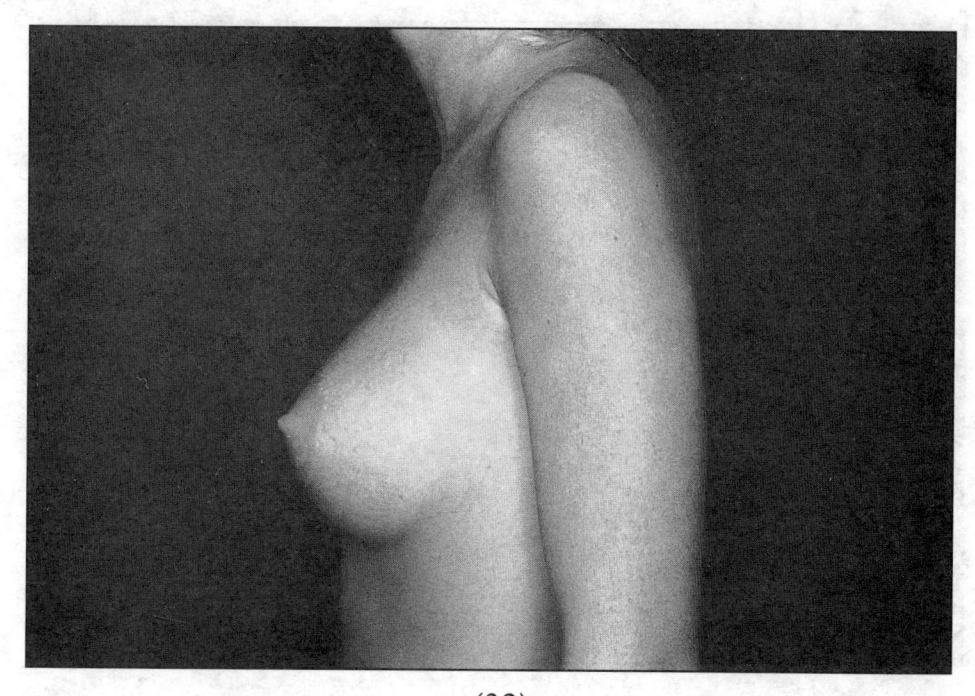

(32)
After

Photographs courtesy of Garth Fisher, M.D.

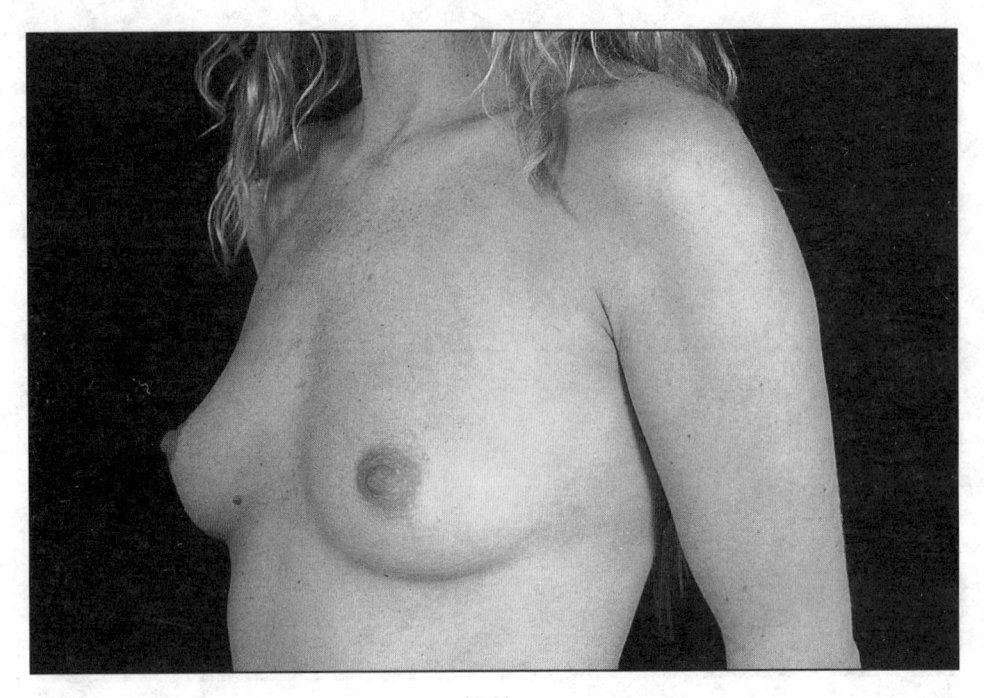

(33)
Breast implants
Before

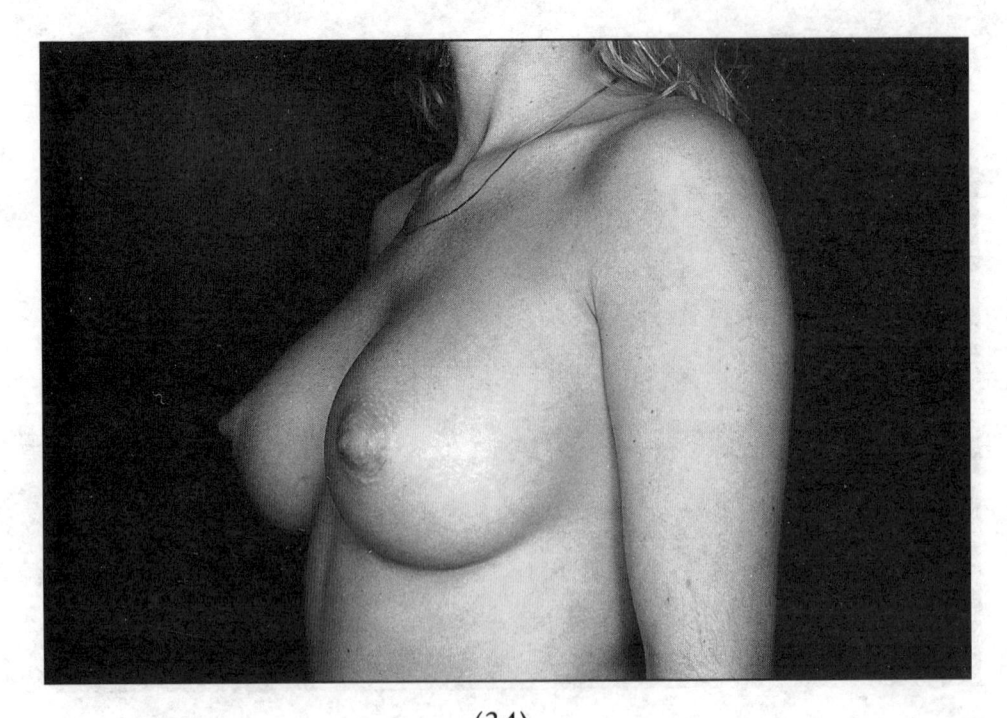

(34)
After

Photographs courtesy of Garth Fisher, M.D.

Husbands And Wives Do It

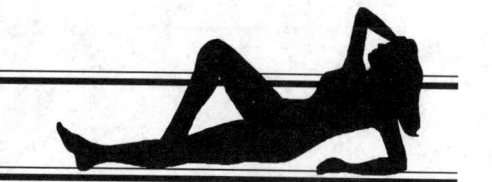

The latest rage in cosmetic surgery is not any one procedure but the fact that husbands and wives are having facelifts together. They make an exciting adventure about the procedure and start to plan a good six months in advance. In most cases the wife goes first and the husband follows the second day. It seems that the reason for the doctor's wait on the husband is because male cosmetic surgical patients don't want to stay in bed at all and get very anxious just laying around. They feel they should be doing work or be on the golf course. No problem, however, with the wives ... they enjoy the pampering.

Occasionally, a couple will choose different doctors and in that case they can arrange for surgery on the same day.

Why a different doctor? Once they have had the consultations by at least three qualified doctors, it is a matter of personal feelings on how comfortable or how one relates to the doctor. A woman and a man may not feel that same "trust" in the same doctor. And doctors understand that. And, as mentioned in FOR MEN ONLY, the procedure is different for men. Some doctors have more experience on men than others.

Husbands and wives usually take this time to make a vacation out of the experience. They seldom tell friends and most friends would not even suspect — they both look so good they just blame it on the Southern California weather. But if only the wife looked so good, they would know.

Couples usually find some excuse to do it. The most common is a wedding anniversary or a high school or college reunion. Many husbands decide to do it just to keep up with the wife.

The most important thing to remember when preparing for a facelift, just like any major party or social function, you need to plan. Give yourself plenty of recuperation time. At least one month for all swelling and bruising to have completely disappeared. If you are planning an outdoor affair soon after your lift, be sure to include a brimmed hat as part of your wardrobe for both of you.

Every couple that has been to The Hidden Garden have been more than ecstatic with the results.

Very often this "affair" becomes their special secret.

For Men Only

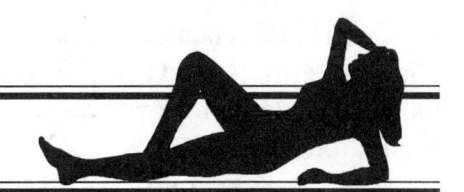

Seven years ago, just after The Hidden Garden was opened, I got a call from a gentleman inquiring as to the services offered at our hideaway. He specifically mentioned that he liked the idea of a hideaway rather than a hotel or going home with a nurse. He inquired about our medium priced rooms, our transportation arrangements (he did not want a limo, "Limo's draw attention") and was happy to hear we used a black Mercedes with tinted windows (very common in Beverly Hills). When I asked him if it were for his wife, he said that it was for himself. "You do take men, don't you, all rooms are private, aren't they?" He continued to tell me that he is a known star on Knots Landing and this was/is to be kept very private. He even reserved under a false name.

When I hung up, I was a little surprised. Somehow I just never thought about facelifts and men. Don't ask me why. I knew men did it. But, ever so rarely.

Not so today. Twenty-five percent of the guests at The Hidden Garden are men. Actors, T.V. personalities, newscasters, weathermen, businessmen, CEO's, attorneys, college professors, movie directors, statesmen, princes, rock stars, movie stars, movie producers, doctors, husbands, and many more. One male guest has been to The Hidden Garden five times in five years. Each summer doing something to improve his looks.

A wonderful husband and wife team just checked out this past weekend. They are celebrating 25 years of marriage. The wife will be back next month for her surgery, the husband went first. I saw his "before" pictures (a large turkey neck, baggy eyes) and without a doubt, he lost ten years. In ten days he looks ten years younger, a common reality with a Facelift.

Another husband and wife couple stayed with us for one full week and then went on to visit the other parts of California for the remainder of their California vacation. He had a facelift, she did not. They were from the South and he was with his company for a long time. Looking tired, looking older, he was being treated that way by his colleagues. He did not feel tired or old, he wanted to maintain his image and his job (like many men who have had the surgery).

Just yesterday a gentleman called and inquired about our hideaway. After answering all the usual questions, he quietly asked, "Do you get a lot of men?" When I responded "of course, twenty-five percent of our guests today are men," I wasn't sure whether his response was one of disappointment (he wasn't the first male) or of relief (there were other men doing it, too).

Men are getting into the act. And why not? You feel good, why not look as good as you feel?

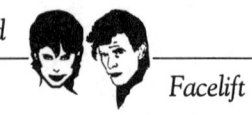

Steve C. visits us every year. A delightful guest, we have his favorite room ready for him for one week early in December. He has himself on a "maintenance" program, doing something each year. One time eyes, the next year a forehead lift, then a little liposuction. At fifty, Steve looks wonderful and will always look wonderful, not just for Christmas, but for the rest of his life. He believes in yearly "touch-ups."

Men always seem to have an edge over women, and here again, with plastic surgery they do as well. No one ever suspects that a man will have a facelift. It's just not conceivable in the real world. Men will drop ten years, look terrific and their co-workers will just attribute it all to his wonder vacation or the Southern California weather. How lucky men are!

What can men do to improve their looks? Lots!

EYES: A major improvement may be attained when eyelid surgery on men is performed. When loose skin develops around the upper and lower eyelids, and when fatty deposits develop under the lower lids, bulging and protrusions are accentuated, creating that tired and sad look. The incisions are made in the skin folds of the eyelids, so natural they are virtually impossible to notice. While healing, it is very important to wear sunglasses and a wide brimmed hat to protect the new incision from any sun damage.

FACELIFTS: Men become wrinkled about ten years later than women. The facial skin texture for men is very different than a woman's. It's thicker and for this reason it is extremely important for men to select not only an experienced doctor, but one who is experienced with male facelifts. Because of the male facial hair, the cutting area and therefore scars must be carefully hidden at the edge of the beard just in front of the ear, and just behind the ears. Large amounts of excessive skin from the neck area is removed, resulting in a more refined, slender neck. No more excessive skin rolling over the collar. A facelift results in a thinner, more youthful appearance.

For the first month after surgery, it is important to wear wide brimmed hats to protect those new little scars from the sun.

The improvement is incredible and may be enjoyed in ten days to two weeks after surgery.

BROW LIFTS: "Excessive" upper eyelid skin is often the result of the relaxation of the eyebrows and sometimes the forehead, as well. When this happens, a "brow lift" is necessary to remove skin just above the brows which will improve the drooping of the brows. This procedure is very successful with men because men usually have numerous forehead wrinkles in which to hide the scars. And in a very short time, most scars will fade and be totally impossible to see. After ten days to two weeks a vast improvement may be seen, a more rested and youthful appearance.

EARS: Men are often troubled with protruding ears, elongated lobes, or overly large shaped ears. "Otoplasty" is the name for this surgery. Incisions are made along the back of the ear to expose the ear cartilage. Depending on the problem, some of this cartilage may be removed or repositioned. The incision behind the ear is sutured for several days. These sutures are removed in seven to ten days. Eyeglasses may be worn after this time. The amount of improvement will depend on the extent of the surgery.

CHEEK AUGMENTATION may be suggested by a plastic surgeon if a more balanced face can be achieved by the implanting of sterile surgical material just in front of the existing cheekbone. Cheek implants are often used to improve the results of a facelift. The look to achieve is a very natural one.

CHIN AUGMENTATION AND REDUCTION are popular cosmetic surgery procedures for men.

Many men have a small chin or a chin that recedes. Building up this type of chin can dramatically improve the facial profile by creating a more prominent jaw line. Using a small incision either inside the mouth or just underneath the chin, the surgeon secures sterile surgical material (similar to the tissue texture of the chin) in front of the jawbone. This procedure will bring out the chin. This implant becomes totally unnoticeable very quickly and will look very natural in two to four weeks.

Chin reduction surgery involves the removal of excess bone from the "chin button" area. When a too long jawbone exists, creating an excessive chin protrusion, this procedure can give the entire profile a more aesthetic balance.

DOUBLE CHIN REDUCTION is accomplished when the problem is not the chin but rather the collection of skin, excessive amounts of fat and skin, under the chin down to the neck. This removal of fat and skin from under the chin is called a "submental lipectomy." This procedure is often part of a full facelift or may be part of a chin reduction or augmentation. The new look will give the face a thinner, more youthful appearance within weeks after surgery.

NOSE surgery, interestingly, is not as popular with men as with women. Most men will only accept a refinement of the nose rather than a complete "new" nose. Because of former nose injuries or breathing problems, men will consider a nose surgery. The nose is associated with "character" and men can carry and look good with "character" noses.

LIPOSUCTION OF THE WAIST area is a very popular procedure. Hundreds of men have resorted to this surgery after trying desperately to reduce the waistline "roll." One 42-year-old male guest at the hideaway agreed to have this surgery after four years of working out and dieting. He had a perfect body everywhere else. This procedure is very simple and takes but an hour or less. The doctor removes fat from the area concerned. The area is wrapped securely for several days and then an adjustable binder may be used for an additional week or two until all swelling is gone. Total results can be seen in four to six weeks. This liposuction procedure is popular with our aging movie stars who want to maintain their youthful figures.

CHEST IMPLANTS, although not common, seem to be popular with men who don't like to exercise or who just don't have the time. Silicone blocks are inserted under the skin. The size depends on the individual. Once implanted, they are soft to the touch, very natural, very real. One can go out in public within a day.

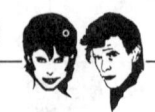

CHEST REDUCTION for men is not so uncommon. This condition is called "gynecomastia" or womanlike breasts. The most common cause is fat. But a chemical imbalance of the liver from the excessive use of alcohol, marijuana and anabolic steroids used in bodybuilding can cause the development of breasts. Liposuction is the procedure to remove this excess fatty tissue.

CALF IMPLANTS, made of the same material as the chest implants, silicone, require more recuperation time. One must stay "off your feet" for several days. However, the results are very dramatic and successful.

BUTT TUCKS, rare, but available, are performed on men who "just want to look good in tight jeans." Although this procedure may not last like other cosmetic procedures, it is very effective when performed. Recover time is at least one week of no sitting.

PENAL IMPLANTS and extensions — this is not a taboo topic. The American Board of Urology can refer experienced doctors in your area. We talk about and even show pictures of women's breasts and breast implants. Why can't men have the equal space to be informed on a very common plastic surgery procedure. A penal implant can change the life of a man, just as breast implants can for a woman.

HAIR REPLACEMENT, Most men with baldness have no control of the condition. It is hereditary. Your genes determine this. Two successful procedures designed to permanently eliminate the baldness and to evenly distribute the existing hair over the entire scalp are flaps and punch grafts. Scalp reductions and expansion are also used to improve the results achieved with flaps and plugs.

Using one's own hair for flaps and plugs makes it a suitable donor source. This technique and combination of techniques has been perfected at The Beverly Hills Institute of Aesthetic & Reconstructive Surgery by doctors Richard Fleming and Toby Mayer. This "Fleming/Mayer Flap" procedure is performed in three surgery stages. And in most cases you can go back to work within a day or two of each surgery. Because the flap is never totally separated from its blood supply, there is no hair loss. Unlike the plugs, there is no "rows of corn" appearance or change of hair texture.

Punch grafts work best for individuals with minimal hair loss. At least four sessions of 25-100 grafts are necessary. The transplanted hair initially falls out but visible hair growth begins in three to four months. Newer punch graft developments include mini and micro grafts for a natural result.

Be very selective and cautious when investigating treatments for baldness. There are many unethical people promising miracle solutions. Never rely on pictures. Always ask to see and talk to actual patients with similar hair texture and baldness pattern before you make any decision. (See What's "Hot" in Beverly Hills).

Nola's Note: With all surgical procedures it is necessary to abstain from sex for the first 48 hours after surgery.

We maintain our cars, we remodel our homes, why not maintain our looks? "As mother nature keeps ticking away, no matter how well we take care of ourselves, some of us need to stay on top of the situation." (M., 50, facelift, browlift, eyes, liposuction)

Face The Risk

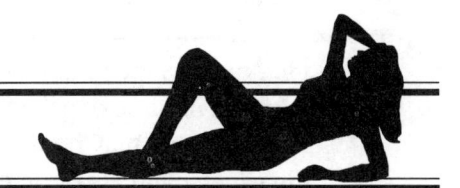

A certain degree of anxiety and apprehension is normal with plastic surgery as with any surgery. However, severe pain is very, very rare. Discomfort is usually the feeling.

Whenever we have a surgery we must weigh the risks. Plastic Surgery procedures, like any surgery, may have its complications although *it is rare*. These risks are another good reason to be sure you have selected a Board Certified, experienced Surgeon.

The main risk in all procedures is the type of anaesthesia used. When properly administered, the anaesthesia used today is so well perfected, side effects are minimal.

The American Association of Nurse Anesthetists have helped the lay person by explaining these two forms of anesthesia as such:

General Anesthesia

Expected Result:	Total unconscious state, possible placement of a tube into the windpipe.
Technique:	Drug injected into the bloodstream, or breathed into the lungs, or by other routes.
Risks:	Mouth or throat pain, hoarseness, injury to mouth or teeth, awareness under anesthesia, injury to blood vessels, aspiration, pneumonia.

Intravenous Regional Anesthesia with Sedation

Expected Result:	Temporary loss of feeling and/or movement of a limb.
Technique:	Drug injected into veins of arm or leg while using a tourniquet.
Risks:	Infection, convulsions, persistent numbness, residual pain, injury to blood vessels.

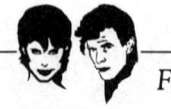

ASK: What are the surgical risks? (And listen!)

1. Hematomas are probably the most frequent complication. Two out of every one hundred patients might experience this small collection of blood underneath the skin of the face. A hematoma may be due to high blood pressure, coughing, twisting ones neck and talking excessively. If at home, do not panic. Apply ice and call your doctor. A hematoma will not ruin you facelift result. It will only slow down your healing time.

2. Hair loss which usually results from direct tension along the suture line is very rare and usually very minimal and only temporary.

3. Bleeding or loss of excessive amounts of blood. More and more surgery patients give one pint of their own blood before surgery to prepare for this occurrence.

4. Scars. These can usually be surgically repaired six to eight weeks after surgery.

5. Bruises are common. The more delicate the surgeon's hands and the healthier the patient, the less bruising occurs. A careful diet on the pre-op days, with no aspirin, no smoking, and no alcohol, all help decrease bruises. This you can control.

6. Infection is very rare, and can be easily treated with an antibiotic.

7. Numbness around the incision areas is common but improves with time.

8. Allergic reactions to the anaesthesia, such as an upset stomach, is only temporary.

9. Poor healing often due to high blood pressure or the use of aspirin products or smoking before surgery—this can be a problem!.

10. Partial facial paralysis or nerve damage is incredibly rare and usually feeling is restored within a month.

11. Abnormal contour of the face or surgical area.

12. Possible distortion of the ears.

13. Dry eyes due to excessive swelling caused by eyes being partially open during surgery, heals within a day or two.

14. With eyelid surgery, abnormal folding-in or folding-out of the eyelids can be repaired with simple exercise. Temporary inflammation of the cornea or interference with the tears drainage can be easily helped with an eye lubricant.

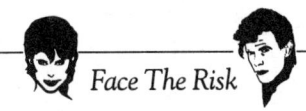

15. Chemical face peels on more olive complexions can result in a much lighter color than the adjacent untreated areas and it may take several months for the skin to blend, but make-up can be successfully used until then.

16. Breast implants have probably the most complications. Changes in the nipple sensation, although usually only temporary can occur. Capsular contracture, unevenness and excessive scar tissue, are the most common complication of breast augmentation although the "new saline implant," has recorded less incidence of this nature.

Nola's Note: It is most important with breast implants to get a yearly mammograph and breast exam. Breast implants do not cause cancer.

Before surgery the doctor will have you sign a "Consent Form" that will make a statement something like this: There is a risk of permanent injury and death associated with all medical and surgical procedures...no guarantee has been made...there are risks involved in the administration of anesthesia...etc.

Read that consent form carefully. If you are in the hands of an experienced, qualified plastic surgeon, you will feel comfortable signing such a form.

One must also understand that it is possible to be unhappy with the result of plastic surgery. Perhaps there is an insufficient amount of wrinkle removal or even an excessive amount. Personality changes and mental difficulties may follow a surgery even when the operation has been a cosmetic success.

A competent surgeon will not recommend an elective cosmetic surgery if you have certain health problems. *At your initial consultation, you should not hide any medical problem.* Be sure to tell the doctor if you have chronic mastitis, diabetes, high blood pressure, any heart, lung, kidney or liver disorder or any serious psychiatric disorder or if you take any medications or are using recreational drugs. And please tell the doctor if you think you might be pregnant!

And *your real age!*

"Health isn't defined by the absence of a few unpleasant physical symptoms. It means being fully alive with vitality, passion, loving and enthusiasm."[8]

Be Prepared
What Can I Do To Prepare Myself For This Surgery?

To ensure quick recovery and the best results from your surgery, thoughtful preparation is essential.

There is a definite difference after surgery with Hidden Garden guests who have taken the time to prepare their bodies, who have made the effort to understand the procedures and who have allowed healing time. They know what to expect, and they are "patient," relaxed patients.

The day you make your surgery date be sure you make reservations for "aftercare." This relieves the burden of friends or a family member to care for you especially since most friends don't know what to expect or what to do. This will be a great relief to you just knowing that you are being cared for by a qualified person. If there are no after care hideaways in your area, arrange for a nurse—*with plastic surgery experience*—to stay with you that first night.

Next, prepare your list of shopping goodies for the first week to ten days post-op. You don't want to be marketing during this time. See the Cookbook recipes for soups and meals to prepare ahead and freeze. Be sure to read and follow the "foods to eat" and "not to eat." Get a note pad and make a list of foods 1) to have on hand, 2) to be prepared. Don't leave things to the last minute. Set a shopping schedule especially if you plan to work up to the day of surgery.

Now think about you and how you can get your body in the very best health for the surgery. Remember, your body is your number one investment.

Ros, 59, spent two weeks before her surgery skiing in Vail, Colorado. She ate carefully and skied a few hours every day. She arrived to surgery a glowing example of health. She says she could "feel the fresh air in her blood." Rosaline went into a six hour surgery—face, eyes, nose, and a breast lift—and came out without a bruise. She healed so quickly that she snuck-out of The Hidden Garden and went shopping on Rodeo Drive. I passed her as she was standing on a corner waiting for the light to change with two huge Nieman Marcus shopping bags just five days post-op.

Nola's Note: **THIS RE-PRINT SHOULD BE READ SEVERAL TIMES!**

What It's Vital to Know Before Your Operation[9]

Each year, tens of thousands of Americans undergo surgery. Fortunately, the vast majority of these operations are successful. Yet several factors—all at least partly avoidable—do sometimes conspire against doctors and patients, resulting in needless pain, longer-than-normal recovery periods and even fatalities.

KEYS TO SAFER SURGERY

- **Maintain a positive mental attitude.** A patient's attitude affects the outcome of surgery almost as much as the surgeon's skill. Many times I've seen terminally ill patients defy the odds and recover fully after a difficult surgery. In contrast, patients with conventionally curable conditions may succumb in surgery—simply because they convince themselves they are doomed.

Key to a speedy recovery: A determination to get out of bed as soon as possible and return to a normal life-style.

Patients who just lie in bed following surgery suffer more complications and stay sicker longer than those who resolve to get back on their feet as soon as possible. The longer you remain in bed following surgery, the greater your risk of suffering a chest infection or a deep vein thrombosis (DVT), a potentially fatal disorder if a clot in the leg breaks off and makes its way to the lungs.

Helpful: Imagine yourself coming through surgery with flying colors and then boasting to friends that you had one of the speediest recoveries on record.

- **Stay physically fit.** Five-mile jogs and strenuous weight-training sessions are *not* necessary. But, being in shape does reduce the risk of infection and complications resulting from surgery.

Physical fitness also shortens the time needed for recovery—sometimes dramatically. Of course, if you need emergency surgery, there's no time for physical conditioning. But if surgery can safely be postponed for a few weeks, use that time to start an exercise regimen. Do aerobic and strength training. Ask your surgeon to recommend any specific exercises that might prove helpful.

Example: Sit ups and leg lifts strengthen the stomach muscles, thereby reducing the risk of hernia following abdominal surgery.

Be sure to inform your surgeon beforehand of any physical limitation or health problem that might complicate surgery. If you catch a cold or flu just prior to your operation, phone your doctor to ask if you should postpone the procedure.

- **Maintain proper nutrition.** Recovery following surgery is a complex process involving tissue repair, replacement of blood and other body fluids, and the fighting of infection.

Poor nutrition hampers the body's ability to perform these functions, placing patients at risk not only of a prolonged recovery, but also of muscle loss, kidney failure and other potentially serious complications. *Especially important:*

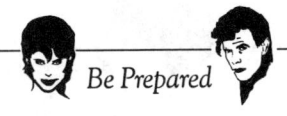

- *For blood replacement:* Iron, vitamin B12 and folate.

- *For prevention of bruising/bleeding:* Vitamin C and vitamin K.

- *For tissue repair:* Zinc.

- *For immunity:* Copper.

- *For prevention of post-surgery constipation:* Dietary fiber.

Bottom line: If you believe your diet is lacking in these nutrients, ask your doctor to recommend a daily multivitamin/mineral supplement.

• **Maintain proper weight.** Being even moderately overweight makes surgery more difficult for surgeons and anesthesiologists, lengthens your recovery period and boosts your risk of complications.

Recent study: Of 500 patients who recently underwent abdominal surgery in an English hospital, those overweight by 30% or more were almost twice as likely to develop serious infections following surgery than were nonobese patients. If you are overweight—and have the time—lose weight before your operation. Avoid crash diets. Lose weight gradually—no more than two pounds a week.

• **Don't smoke.** Smoke retards the healing process and interferes with the action of certain important drugs. Smokers are six times more likely to develop chest infections following abdominal surgery than are nonsmokers.

While four to six weeks of abstinence are needed to curb these risks, giving up cigarettes even for a few days or hours prior to surgery is extremely beneficial.

Background: Tobacco smoke contains carbon monoxide, a substance highly toxic to hemoglobin, the blood protein responsible for transporting oxygen throughout the body. Less healthy hemoglobin means slower healing following surgery. Tobacco smoke also contains nicotine, a powerful stimulant that forces the heart to pump faster and to use more oxygen. Though this extra burden does not ordinarily pose a severe problem, it has been known to cause heart attacks in some surgical patients—especially those who have been smoking for many years.

• **Limit alcohol consumption.** Heavy drinkers—especially those who can "hold their liquor" without becoming visibly drunk—often require more anesthetic than nondrinkers.

This difference poses problems for anesthesiologists who are not forewarned. In addition, heavy drinkers often have nutritional deficiencies that compromise the post-surgery healing process. Finally, heavy drinking irritates the liver, hampering the organ's ability to break down medications and to produce proteins essential to clotting of the blood.

Bottom line: The less you drink, the safer your surgery.

- **Check your medications.** While most prescription drugs can safely be taken up to and during the period of surgery, others may interfere with safe anesthesia or surgery. Consult your surgeon if you are taking insulin, an anticoagulant or steroids. The dose will need adjusting for surgery.

In addition, birth control pills containing estrogen raise the risk of deep vein thrombosis during surgery. The Pill should be avoided for at least four weeks prior to major surgery.

Exception: The so-called "minipill" does not contain estrogen and is safe to use prior to surgery.

- **Secure loose dental work—and repair decayed teeth.** Anesthesia often involves insertion of tubes and instruments into the patient's mouth. If your teeth are loose or badly decayed, or if you have a bridge or other fragile dental work, tell your surgeon well before any surgery.

Danger: Loose teeth or dental work may become lodged in the throat or windpipe, resulting in breathing difficulties. In addition, bacteria present in decayed teeth may spread infection elsewhere in the body following surgery. Cavities should be filled well in advance of surgery.

READY . . . SET . . . GO!!! *60 DAYS PRIOR TO SURGERY:*

- Stop smoking. (At least cut down!)
- Use aspirin or aspirin products only when necessary. (See Doctor John's list).
- Drink 8-10 glasses of water daily.
- Eat high iron foods. (see list)
- Eat high protein foods.
- Eat high potassium foods. (see list)
- Eat low fat foods.
- Cut down on alcoholic drinks.
- Cut down on caffeine.
- Avoid taking any unnecessary medications such as sleeping pills or Valium.
- Stop using recreational drugs.
- If you are under another doctor's care, check to make sure this elective surgery is approved.
- Check to see if you are pregnant.
- Let hair grow wild for new styling later.
- Exercise as usual or at least develop a minimal program.
- Eat healthy foods. Include carbohydrates, protein, fiber. Don't go on any crash diet now, if you eat well and don't overeat, you will probably lose weight. Try to maintain an even weight. You need nutrients for proper healing.
- Take "before" pictures.
- Arrange for your aftercare "Hideaway" or nurse.

Nola's Note: Don't change your life style, just clean it up!

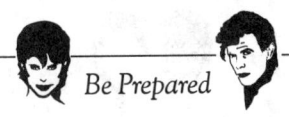

30 DAYS PRIOR TO SURGERY:
- Stop smoking *now!*
- Limit to two glasses of alcohol per day.
- Avoid caffeine - switch to decaf.
- Stop taking *extra* vitamin E and vitamin A (blood thinners).
- Cut down on papaya products (possible blood thinners).
- Do not eat garlic in large amounts (another blood thinner).
- Avoid aspirin and ibuprofen.
- Take a good multiple Vitamin twice a day.
- Eliminate spices, salt (may cause increased swelling after surgery).
- Continue good exercise program to improve blood circulation to the skin.
- Continue to let hair grow for new styling later.
- Get your teeth cleaned and have dental work completed.
- Get your last facial before surgery.

15 DAYS PRIOR TO SURGERY:
- No smoking.
- No caffeine. (Can interfere with medications)
- No alcohol. (Causes bruising, lessens the ability of your body to metabolize medications)
- No aspirin or ibuprofen or aspirin-containing products.
- No recreational or social drug use.
- Take extra Vitamin K if necessary. (Need doctor's prescription.)
- No meat tenderizer or fish oil tablets.
- No Vitamin E.
- No spicy foods. No salt.
- Eat high iron foods.
- No sunbathing or tanning booths.
- No new skin products.
- Avoid people who seem to have the flu or a cold.
- Call to confirm your "Hideaway" stay.
- Take care of financial matters now: pay bills.

10 DAYS PRIOR TO SURGERY:
- Arrange for shopping and recipes to be prepared. (See **The Hidden Garden Cookbook**)
- Arrange for phone calls, etc. "I'm at the Spa; be back in 10 days!"
- Get hair color now.
- Notify your doctor if you develop any cold sores or skin infections.
- Eat high iron foods daily.
- Eat carbohydrates: lots of whole grains, fruits and vegetables.
- Check with your doctor about discontinuing any current medications.
- Take all pre-op tests.
- Give blood to be stored for your surgery if required.

Face surgeries:
- Purchase a scarf and a hat with a large sun brim.
- Purchase a hooded sweatshirt (less conspicuous to walk about in.)
- Purchase a large pair of sunglasses but light in weight.
- Purchase a speaker phone.
- Purchase a child's toothbrush.
- Purchase a pair of large cotton men's pajamas or night shirt (more comfortable than nightgowns.)

Nola's Note: We do not recommend any pullovers, they can catch the earlobes and pull them.

3 DAYS PRIOR TO SURGERY:
- If you think you are pregnant, get tested.
- Shower daily with Dial or Phisoderm.
- Pre-purchase medications.
- Avoid dairy products (seem to increase mucus)
- Avoid citrus fruits (may be too acidic)
- No hair color or tints or bleach.
- If you wear a wig, please notify the Office.
- Select video tapes or listening tapes, old movies, books on tape. (Reading and concentration are difficult after surgery.)
- Arrange for a ride to surgery. Arrange for a ride home from surgery or home from your post-op hideaway.

2 DAYS PRIOR TO SURGERY:
- Pack for Hideaway:
  - Large pair men's pajamas, cotton.
  - Child's toothbrush.
  - Medications.
  - Video tapes or listening tapes, books on tape, etc.
  - Eye glass case or contact lens case or dentures case.
  - Leave reading materials or office work at home.
  - Leave jewelry and all valuables at home.

1 DAY PRIOR TO SURGERY:
- Take a long walk, see a movie or enjoy a concert.
- Eat a nutritious, high protein and high carbohydrate dinner. No salt.
- Drink eight full glasses of water.
- Wash hair with Neutrogena Shampoo or Baby Shampoo or as doctor directed.
- Absolutely:
- No aspirin—causes bleeding.
- No alcohol—causes bruising.

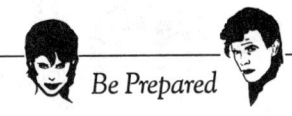

- No dairy—causes delivery of mucous in the stomach.
- No citrus—causes an acid stomach.
- No caffeine—interferes with medication.
- No chocolate—has caffeine.
- No coffee/tea—has caffeine.
- Do not eat or drink after midnight.

It seems the anesthesia has a tendency to do strange things to the stomach acids. This imbalance creates a nauseous feeling after surgery. The dinner before your surgery is very important. Everyone is different, but on the average most guests have no nausea when they follow a very simple day-before menu. The basic principle of this menu is to eat *(not stuff yourself)* high protein, potassium and iron, which is needed for repair and reconstruction of tissues; high carbohydrates for reserved energy for the following "surgery" and fiber for easy digestion and elimination. Our Nurse Elizabeth has a wonderful down-home recipe for the pre-op dinner: eat something sweet with real sugar for dessert: apple pie! Blueberry tart! Sugar coats the stomach lining and gives energy. And some fat. Fat helps the body absorb medications into your system, especially the antibiotic and other medication you will be taking the next day.

A "health food" inspired friend went into surgery with a dinner of peanut butter with mashed banana on multigrain bread, a large bean and spinach salad, and two large glasses of water. Dessert - apple pie.

Actually, if you look at her meal carefully, she did okay. Peanut butter = protein/fat. Bananas = potassium. Bread = carbohydrate. Water = water. Salad = iron and fibre. Apple pie = sugar.

DAY OF SURGERY
- Wear hooded sweat outfit or warm-up outfit that buttons or zips up front.
- Wear comfortable, flat shoes but not sandals or sling backs.
- Do not wear make-up.
- Do not wear panty hose and heels.
- Do not eat or drink anything after midnight.
- Do not wear jewelry or bring valuables to surgery.
- If you wear contacts or dentures or glasses, bring the appropriate case with you.

RELAX.

DOCTOR JOHN'S ASPIRIN LIST[10]

All patients anticipating surgery must stop the use of *all sources* of aspirin. Aspirin is a very strong anticoagulant which causes profound bleeding problems in normal individuals. Therefore, you must stop taking aspirin and all aspirin containing products for 2-weeks before surgery and *2-weeks after surgery*. The following are only a few of many aspirin containing compounds:

Advil	Cama-Inlay Tabs	Ibuprofen	Persisti
Alka Seltzer	Choracol Capsules	Indocin	Robaxisal
Anacin	Clinorll	Measurin	Sine-Aid
Anaprox	Congespirin	Midol	Sine-Off
A.P.C.	Cope	Monacet with	SK-Compound
Ascodeen-30	Coricidin	Codeine	Capsules
Ascriptin	Darvon Compound	Motrin	Stendin
Aspirin	Dristan	Naprosyn	Stero-Darvon
Aspirin	Duragesic	Norgesic	w/A.S.A.
Suppositories	Esotrin	Nuprin	Supac
Bayer Aspirin	Emprazil	Percodan	Synalgos Capsules
BC Powders	Empirin	Percogesic	Synalgos D.C.
Buff-a-Comp	Equageslc	Pabirin Buffered	Tolectin
Buffadyne	Excedrin	Tabs	Triaminicin
Bufferin	Feldene	Panalgesic	Vanquish
Butalbital	Fiorinal	Pepto-Bismol	Zomax

Following are some aspirin containing topical medications to be avoided:

Absorbent Rub	Baumodyhne	Icy Hot	Rumarub
Absorbine Arthritic	Ben Gay	Infra-Rub	Sloan's
Absorbine Jr.	Braska	Lini-Balm	Soltice
Act-On Rub	Counterpain Rub	Mentholatum	SPD
Analbalm	Dencorub	Musterole	Stimurub
Analgesic Balm	Doan's Rub	Neurabaim	Surin
Antiphiogistine	Emul-O-Baim	Oil-O-Sol	Yager's Liniment
Arthralgen	End-Ake	Omega Oil	Zemo Liquid
Aspercreme	Exocaine	Panalgesic	Zemo Ointment
Banalg	Heet	Rid-A-Pain	

If you must take something for headache, menstrual cramps or other aches and pains, you may take Tylenol (as directed) for the two weeks prior to and after your surgery.

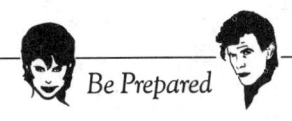

IRON RICH FOODS

Iron is needed to manufacture healthy red blood cells. Minimum daily requirements are: 10 mg/day for men and postmenopausal women; 18 mg./day for menstruating women.

Include citrus fruits and juices with your meals for more efficient absorption of the iron. Also, cooking in cast iron cookware significantly increases your intake of iron.

MEATS

Beef, 4 oz.	4.2 mg.
Chicken, 4 oz.	1.1 mg.
Turkey, 4 oz.	4.6 mg.
Clams, 4 oz.	8.4 mg.
Oysters, 4 oz.	6.8 mg.
Sardines, 4 oz.	3.2 mg.
Pork, 4 oz.	1.3 mg.
Lamb, 4 oz.	2.5 mg.
Liver, 4 oz. (beef)	9.4 mg.
Liver, 4 oz. (chicken)	9.7 mg.
Egg, 1 medium	1.0 mg.

FRUITS

Apricots, dried, ½ cup	1.3 mg.
Avocado, ½ medium	1.0 mg.
Prune juice, 1 cup	10.0 mg.
Raisins, ½	2.5 mg.

BREAD AND GRAINS

40% Bran flakes 1 cup	1.0 mg.
Raisin Bran, 1 cup	9.0 mg.
Oatmeal, 1 cup	1.6 mg.
Cream of Wheat, 1 cup	7.9 mg.

VEGETABLES

Artichoke (1)	1.6 mg.
Beans, cup cooked	
(garbanzo)	3.4 mg.
(kidney)	1.9 mg.
(lima)	1.8 mg.
Brussel sprouts (6-7)	1.4 mg.
Chard, swiss, cooked	1.2 mg.
Dandelion greens, ½ cup cooked	2.0 mg.
Lentils, ½ cup cooked	2.0 mg.
Peas, sweet ½ cup	1.6 mg.
Peas, blackeyed, ½ cup	1.8 mg.
Potato, baked, 1 medium	.7 mg.

NUTS

Almonds, ¼ cup	1.5 mg.
Cashews, ¼ cup	1.3 mg.
Walnuts, ¼ cup	1.0 mg.

MISCELLANEOUS

Molasses, 1 tbsp.	.9 mg.
Yeast, dried Brewers, 2 tbs.	2.7 mg.

Hiding Out

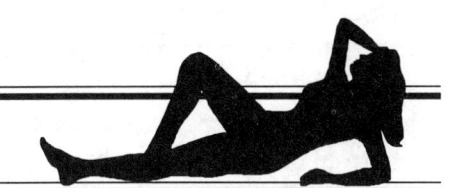

Linda (F, 53, face/eyes) was out of surgery on time on a Monday and I picked her up after the usual restful time in recovery. During the ride to The Hidden Garden, she quietly asked, "How do I look? ... I'm having a dinner party on Saturday."

Actually Linda didn't look bad: her eyes were a puffy deep shade of mauve, her cheeks/jowls were not badly swollen, her neck was only slightly bruised. The bandages around her head, turban like, made her look like a very serious person from some new religious group.

"Well, people pay a lot of money for that color eye shadow," I said.

Linda went on to tell me how her girlfriend looked great from the very first day, and after just four days was shopping on Rodeo Drive. After all, that's one reason she chose her friend's doctor and followed his instructions so carefully. What Linda and many other cosmetic surgery patients don't realize is the fact that everyone heals differently. They heal at a different rate. Age and overall health are major factors. Some people are "bruisers." Some people retain water. Some surgeries are more involved. Bone structure and skin texture all add to the complexity of the healing process.

Another Hidden Garden guest complained about her swelling and bruising. After her first facelift, she just went home and couldn't understand why she didn't feel as good this time. Her first facelift was ten years before at age fifty-five. One's body is just not the same after ten years.

It is very true the earlier you start to take care of the "aging face," the less trauma there is to the body and there is less recuperation time.

If you know your body, you can plan better for your aftercare.

There is rarely pain with cosmetic surgery. Depending on the surgery, most guests are comfortable with a mild pain medication or extra strength Tylenol. The biggest complaint we get is having to sleep on one's back and being uncomfortable wearing the head dressing. "It's like sleeping with your hair in curlers and I haven't done that for thirty years!"

Most doctors insist on two-three nights in an aftercare facility because of the *unknown side effects of an anaesthesia* on your body. Aftercare facilities are designed to foresee and handle problems. They have experienced staff trained in plastic surgery procedures.

Going home with a private duty nurse at $25 per hour for the first day can cost about $500, then you still need meals and housekeeping. Aftercare facilities, such as The Hidden Garden, start at $350 a night and include a private room and bath, all meals, transportation and expert nursing care. You are in a supportive and informative atmosphere, not a hospital. The perfect half-way place. Consider such a stay seriously.

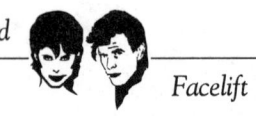

Doctors will require patients to be "elevated," either the upper body or lower or both. A good aftercare facility will provide you, at no extra cost, with an adjustable bed to make you more comfortable. It is very important to draw the bodily fluids away from the surgical area and then there will be much less swelling. If you must go home and cannot afford to rent an adjustable bed, try taking the bottom cushion of your living room sofa and placing it between the bed mattress and box spring. Add pillows beneath your knees, if you have had lower body work or back pain. This trick helps but is not as good as having an adjustable bed. The difference in comfort and recovery time is very noticeable.

A pillow behind your head will push your head forward and chin down. Use a neck roll or make one by rolling a bath towel and placing it under your neck. Do not use a pillow. The tip of your chin should be pointing towards the ceiling, NOT towards your feet.

If you go home, remember that emergencies are rare, but problems can occur.

CALL THE DOCTOR IMMEDIATELY:

1. If your temperature is over 101 degrees.

2. If you notice excessive swelling on one side of your face.

3. In case of excessive bleeding.

4. In case of persistent vomiting.

5. Any time you feel something might be seriously wrong.

POST-OP DAYS:

Doctors seem to slide through the post-op days very quickly. The reason is very simple. Doctors don't want to scare people away or make a big issue about the surgery and everyone heals differently. General anesthesia patients will find themselves moving slower, losing the ability to concentrate. Patients will experience headaches, be very thirsty, and be more tired.

For two weeks after surgery:

NO SMOKING
NO SALT
NO CAFFEINE

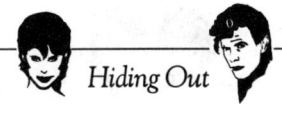

While on antibiotics:

    No raw meat or chicken

    No sushi

    Eat yogurt with the live lactobacillus culture

Nola's Note: Antibiotics kill off all the good bacteria in your system.

GENERAL GUIDELINES:

Face and Head Surgery Patients: Face, eyes, browlift patients all need to have the head elevated for several days.

No driving for five to seven days. To begin with, the anesthesia stays within your body for several days. Light-headedness or dizziness is not uncommon. You don't want to be driving and experience these feelings. It is important not to turn your neck after a facelift since this can strain the muscle work done to complete your necklift.

Nola's Note: California law actually says that you can't drive for thirty days following general anesthesia.

Face surgery patients are discouraged from chewing. Stay totally away from any: nuts and seeds (even raspberries), jams with tiny seeds, corn on the cob, whole apples, pears and peaches, hard candy, caramels, beef jerky, crusty bread, raw carrots, celery, broccoli stems, lettuces, meat and chicken (unless ground or finely chopped) and fish with bones.

    No gum chewing.

    No excessive talking!

    Use a speaker phone.

    Brush your teeth with a child's tooth brush.

    No bending to tie shoes, etc.

    Avoid sun or sitting in a hot area (i.e., the beach, a tennis match).

    Avoid all exercises that will build up a "sweat."

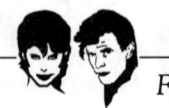

Wear loose eye glasses (or tape to forehead), avoid contacts.

Eyes will be sensitive to the sunlight. Wear sunglasses.

Cover all scars with sunblock.

Wear wide brimmed hats.

Avoid plants and flowers that might make you sneeze.

Avoid all spicy foods.

Do not wear earrings for two to three weeks.

Facials should be avoided for at least 6 weeks, then only a gentle cleaning is allowed.

Do not wear tight necked T-shirts or turtlenecks for at least three weeks. Be careful pulling clothes over your head! Chemical peels require a 6 month period of sun abstinence with the daily use of a Sunscreen.

Breast Surgery Patients: Do not use your arms. Therefore do not: drive, lift, reach, or carry anything, and do not comb or brush one's hair for three to ten days.

Lipsuction and Tummy Tuck Surgery Patients: Eat foods high in potassium and iron. Tummy tuck patients need to have their legs and upper body elevated. Walking up and down stairs will be difficult.

Eyelid Surgery Patients: Use cold compresses for the first 24-48 hours. (Apply 4 x 4 pads soaked in ice water then squeezed of excessive water, or crushed ice wrapped in a baggie or washcloth. Change every 20 minutes. Direct ice is *too* cold.) With eyelid surgery, some degree of blurred vision is expected for two to three days. This is usually due to the ointment used (to prevent dryness) and the swelling that develops.

All Surgery Patients: See **The Hidden Garden Cookbook** and **The Hollywood Facelift Diet**.

The Hollywood Facelift Diet and the following **Hidden Garden Cookbook** recipes are a very big help to those at home. Your post-op diet is extremely important for healing. It is important to eat foods high in protein, high in potassium and low in sodium. Liquid to soft diets are prescribed for almost all surgeries. Remember, the stomach is not ready to digest *solid* foods for the first 24-48 hours, no matter how hungry you may feel.

Medications of any kind have a tendency to irritate the stomach. It's best to be very careful of what you eat and take it very slowly. The Hidden Garden nurses start the patient with jello and thinly sliced fresh bananas. The sugar in the jello coats the stomach and the banana is high in potassium to help with fluid loss/dehydration.

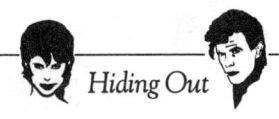

Calories are necessary for healing, BUT pick and choose good calories: eggs, because they are high in protein and soft, are a good source at this time, especially egg whites. Also, doctors want some sugar in the diet, sugars in the form of fructose: fruits like watermelon, cantaloupe, mango, pineapple, and kiwi. Avoid diet drinks, doctors prefer the no caffeine soft drinks with real sugar.

Caffeine interferes with the medications given at this time, and citrus foods can upset the stomach. So, *no caffeine* and *no citrus fruits* until all prescribed medications are finished and, of course, *no alcohol.*

Drink at least eight glasses of water daily. Your liver has been overloaded with medications and your body needs to be cleansed.

HOW LONG DO YOU NEED TO HIDE OUT?

How long you need to hide out depends on how much surgery you have. Naturally, the more you do the longer it will take to spring back to your old self again. Depending on your swelling and bruises, most face and eyelid surgeries can go anywhere one week after their surgery.

Doctors discourage *all* surgery patients who have been given a general anesthesia from driving themselves for five to ten days. The body's reflexes are slower and driving can be dangerous. Eyes, after all surgeries, tend to be watery and very sensitive to the sunlight, even with sunglasses. Check with your doctor and use your common sense.

Flying should be avoided for five to ten days, depending on the surgery. Nose surgery patients usually are discouraged from flying for at least ten days.

A male guest at The Hidden Garden was given permission to fly home several days after surgery. While in the air, he looked up to see what "red oil" was dripping on his shirt. He immediately realized that the plane was not dripping, he was. He had started to bleed profusely. The cabin pressure can cause a scab to "pop" off and for bleeding to occur. Our guest was very calm. Not to say the same for his seat partner or the flight attendant. The pilot immediately turned the plane around and it returned to LAX. Our guest's doctor and nurse were waiting at the airport gate for his return. This is a true story!!

Nola's Note: Check with your doctor. Changes in the cabin air pressure can cause not only your ears to "pop" but the sudden hemorrhaging of surgical incisions.

Going back to work depends on each individual's surgery and you and the doctor need to discuss this carefully.

Contact lenses—ask the doctor.

Sun exposure is prohibited for six weeks to six months depending on the surgery.

"Baths, showers and shampoos are based on each individual's case and your surgeon's approval. Make-up can be applied once the surgeon has given you the OK. Each person heals differently and at a different rate—so please check, there are no rules! Tissue healing is an individual characteristic and varies from patient to patient."[11]

Our **Hollywood Facelift Diet** helps your system to return to normal and enhances proper nutrition. It is very important at this time to build new tissues, renew blood supply and reduce swelling and bruising as soon as possible. You will expect to feel tired up to four weeks after surgery.

For plastic surgery in general:

1. Dressings will be removed in 2-5 days.

2. Swelling and skin discoloration subside within 1-2 weeks.

3. Tightness and numbness varies with each individual.

4. Itchiness will develop at the incision site, about 5-7 days.

5. Hair shampooing, 3-6 days. Color 4 weeks. Perm 6 weeks.

6. Shower and baths, 3-6 days.

7. Sutures are removed anywhere from 3 days to 2 weeks.

8. Scar tissue is pink at first. Scars will lighten in color within 3-6 months. Scars tend to flatten and blend after 4-5 weeks.

9. Light exercise, walking, stretching, 2 weeks after surgery. Resume your normal exercise program after 4-6 weeks.

10. Make-up can be gently applied by day 5. Lipstick immediately!

Remember, it's like remodeling your house—it looks worse before it looks better!

To Tell Or Not To Tell

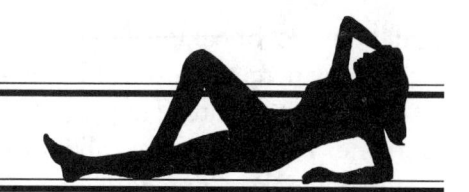

Your surgery is a very personal matter. Some guests have no problem with people knowing. They tell all their friends and can't wait to show-off the results. Huge bouquets of flowers arrive.

Other guests feel it is a private matter, have few visitors if any, often calling home and telling the family how wonderful "the spa" is.

It's a personal decision.

In the olden' days, back in the late 1800's in Paris, women would sneak into the surgeons back door on a Friday, have a "nip and tuck" performed, go to the country to "hideaway" until Monday. They would return very refreshed from the country air and fresh foods—the very same goes on today.

Many women start young and go regularly to their plastic surgeon just like those regular visits to their gynecologist or dentist. A little eye work one time, lipo under the chin the next, browlift, etc., etc., etc. Nothing that would put them out of the social scene too long, therefore, no one would ever guess.

Men, on the other hand, usually don't tell. They'll come from all over the world to Beverly Hills for a facelift, eyelift, liposuction, or chest implants. They stay ten days to two weeks and when they go home, they just tell everyone about their Southern California vacation. Many, many, many *husbands and wives* do just that.

Often you can disguise your new look with a new haircut and color. Get the color done a few days before surgery and a new hairstyle just after the sutures are taken out. Letting your hair grow wild and awful the month before surgery will only help you look better afterwards.

Men usually let their beards grow. After four to six weeks (when all is healed), shave. Most people will associate the new look with just being "clean shaven" again. Many men keep the mustache just for fun!

A lovely Japanese lady had her plan. She left travel brochures around her desk months before her surgery date. Having very short, black hair, she couldn't do much to change her hairstyle, but instead she carefully planned a new wardrobe to distract her co-workers from suspecting. Normally, she wore dark conservative colors and suits. She shopped and found gorgeous vibrant silk shirts in magenta, canary yellow, lime green and hot reds. She arrived back at work with a new wardrobe—it worked!

Nose surgery is very acceptable in today's society. In fact, many nose surgeries are not considered cosmetic. Sneaking in both eyes and a facelift can be done without too much notice, depending on how perceptive your friends are.

Others don't care. They are going to tell and show their new $15,000 face/body to anyone and everyone. They are excited about their new look. "Besides, everyone is doing it." They make a party of it. Several girl friends will have facelifts together at the same time. Often, The Hidden Garden Hideaway feels more like a College Campus Sorority House.

We have a tendency to be too critical of ourselves. We see people as a "picture," a head to toe picture. Even your best friends don't look at every line or skin discoloration. They see you as you. That overall image that makes you, you. An extra large nose, a character nose, may be the only exception.

People form an image of people. My daughter and I wear the same dress size and usually dress very casually, in fact, we share our clothes. Several years ago we both got short, bobbed haircuts. We looked so much alike, my friends mistook me for my daughter—a full twenty-five years younger!

Usually if you plan your surgery with a "good story," you can get away with people not knowing you had surgery. Decorators take trips to Europe, men go on conventions, wives wait for husbands to be out of town.

One guest, a very careful planner, called six weeks in advance and made it clear that she would call us, I was not to call her. Her husband was going on location to Spain. She scheduled her surgery the following morning at 6:30 a.m. and a five-day hideaway stay afterwards. Then days before, when she passed all her tests, she carefully let everyone know that she, too, would go away—to the spa—for a few days. All was under control until the day before . . . her husband's trip got delayed *one* day. (She had to tell him!)

Two months before ski season, Shirley, a psychotherapist, stayed at The Hidden Garden. Her doctor was carefully selected by Shirley after seeing two other plastic surgeons in the Los Angeles area. Seeing Shirley one month after her surgery I couldn't help being curious about her reactions to her new look! After all, who would be more observant than a psychotherapist. We had a wonderful visit. I felt her descriptions were very real and asked her to please put them down on paper.

". . . to tell or not to tell, that is the question."

"A WRINKLE IN TIME"

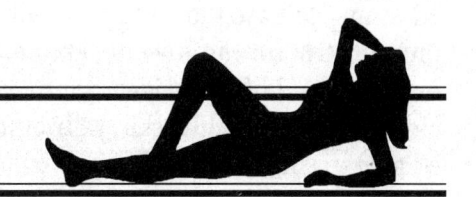

by Shirley C. Geller, Ph.D.

I had never contemplated a facelift until a six-year old boy astutely observed that the folds in my face had increased with time. In my capacity as a clinical psychologist I had first seen this child when he was three. When he returned at age six after not seeing me for three years, he immediately questioned whether I was the Dr. Geller who saw him three years ago. I told him I was. He continued to be unsure of my identity commenting, "You talk like Dr. Geller, you are in Dr. Geller's office but you don't look like Dr. Geller." I told him that maybe the reason I didn't look the way he remembered me was that I had become thinner and was wearing my hair differently. He quickly replied, "Oh, no that isn't it." While running his little fingers over his own face, he replied, "The reason you don't look like Dr. Geller is that you have more wrinks." I was astonished that a six year old child was cognizant of sagging skin.

This led me to think about the newly acquired wrinkles in my face and neck. Most of my life I had focused on professional activities. I had obtained a Ph.D. in psychology, authored a number of research and clinical papers, and most recently become a graduate psychoanalyst. After spending fourteen years in analysis, one day I looked into the mirror, and I came up with a sobering realization. By the time I arrived at the point in my life where my insides were congruent with my outsides, my outsides had begun to deteriorate. I wasn't ready for this. I had thought that reaching middle age would leave me feeling old and living a sedentary life. But neither feeling old nor leading a sedentary life seemed to apply to me. No longer married and with my daughter away at college, I had joined several ski clubs. In my mid-fifties, I found myself jogging, water and snow skiing as well as trekking the Alps and Himalayas. I had lost seventeen pounds, discovered clothes and make-up and was really feeling terrific. My psyche and physique were in good condition, but as my six year old patient had observed, I had more "wrinks."

I began to give some thought to the idea of plastic surgery. One day while passing a plastic surgeon's office, I decided to go in and make an appointment for a consultation. The idea of actually having plastic surgery began to take on the quality of an adventure. I then made appointments with two other surgeons. All three came highly recommended, were members of the American Society of Plastic and Reconstructive Surgeons, and were on teaching staffs of medical schools. I took notes during the consultations. Additionally, I compared and contrasted their suggested procedures, techniques, and fees. Even though I was only interested in removing the wrinkles in the lower portion of my face and neck in the beginning, I ended up with much more. The surgeon I selected suggested a muscle based facelift. Not only would loose skin be removed from my face and neck but the muscle structure in my cheekbone, jawline, and neck region would be tightened. I had read that muscle-based lifts provided the strongest, most effective, longest-lasting results. Furthermore, muscle-layer work, unlike skin tightening alone, rarely needed redoing. My surgeon also recommended an extreme forehead lift and upper eyelid surgery. The former was to correct my sagging eyebrows, as well as decrease eyelid "hooding," and reduce the frown lines in my forehead. A forehead lift involves pulling the skin of the forehead up and suturing it into the front of the skull. The eyelid surgery was for the purpose of removing loose skin in my eyelids. To give a more aesthetically complete look some shaving of the bones above the eyelids plus the removal of small pads of fat in the lower portion of the cheeks were also suggested. Since I viewed having facial plastic surgery as a once in a lifetime venture, I elected to have all of the recommended procedures performed.

Once the procedures and date for surgery had been finalized, I found myself alternately filled with excitement and terror. But my terror took an unusual form. One day while sitting listening to a therapy patient, I found myself growing painfully sleepy. The woman whom I was seeing questioned whether she was boring me. Thank heavens it occurred towards the end of the hour. I apologized. As soon as she left the office, I phoned my internist and detailed my symptoms to him. He questioned me in regard to the food I had earlier eaten. He also asked if I was under any stress. I informed him that I had eaten some low-calorie popcorn an hour before and, "Yes, I was under stress." I told him I had just set the date to have my facelift done. I was scared to death but going to go ahead with it anyway. He then told me that my uncontrollable attack of sleepiness was due to a lowering of blood sugar caused by anxiety, a psycho-physiological stress reaction. The date of my surgery was two months off and here I was, a psychotherapist, falling asleep on patients due to anxiety. For the next two months I adhered to a hypoglycemic diet while at work. I could not risk almost falling asleep on a patient again.

A month before surgery I informed both my adult and child patients I would be having, "some minor cosmetic surgery." I told them I might look slightly different. Since some of my patients already are uncertain about their perceptions of reality, I did not want to add to their confusion. I did not discuss any of my concerns with my patients but only focused on the meaning my surgery had for them. I told them I would be out of the office for two weeks. Another psychologist plus a psychiatrist would be available to handle any emergencies. I would be available to speak with them by phone the second week.

The surgery would be performed in the doctors' office. In the Los Angeles area the plastic surgeons typically perform cosmetic surgery in their office suites. A portion of their suites include an operating room and recovery area. Their offices are located near hospitals in order to handle complications that might arise. Patients may elect to return home following the surgery as long as they have someone to care for them. Or they may choose to go to a private, convalescent facility for cosmetic surgery patients. I chose the latter. While I did not need the elegance and pampering of an exclusive Beverly Hills hideaway, my house was some distance from the doctor's office and he felt it would be prudent to stay in a recovery facility near his office.

About a month before the surgery, a beautifully printed brochure about my convalescent hideaway arrived. The office staff and other tenants in my suite were eager to learn what a guest house for cosmetic surgery patients was like. They envied my being driven from the surgeon's office to the guest house in a Rolls Royce. They also were curious about spa cuisine prepared for people who had limited capacity to chew.

In retrospect, I believe the two strongest emotions I felt in relation to my upcoming surgery were *terror* and *denial*. Terror that someone was going to be pulling on and cutting my skin. Denial that I had signed up for a procedure that would involve some pain and risk.

Eight A.M. Thursday, October 25th, I arrived at the doctor's office. I wrote out a check for the anesthetist, donned a hospital gown, lay down on the operating table and let sublimaze drip into my veins. With classical music playing in the background, the surgeon began drawing a line across the crown of my head, from one ear to another. This was to be the site of the incision for the extreme forehead lift. At that very moment the denial that I had disappeared and the reality that I indeed was having surgery clicked in. I began to experience some panic and thought, "Oh my God, what have I gotten myself into now?" I did not verbalize the full extent of my panic to my doctor. Instead I commented that I was experiencing some anxiety. The surgeon, who like myself is a skier, replied, "don't worry, anxiety is normal. It's just like the anxiety you experience when you are at the top of a black ski run before you come down." After hearing those words I knew I was doomed. For black runs are the most dangerous and difficult of all ski runs. I weakly replied, "but I don't do black runs." The last two thoughts that occurred to me prior to the anesthesia completely taking over were whatever contribution I was going to make to this world I had already made and my will was within plain sight on the desk in my study. My heirs would have no problem finding it.

The next thing I was conscious of was being in the recovery area with the doctor telling me the surgery was over. It took five and a half hours. My head and neck were sheathed in bandages, I was weak and feeling somewhat nauseous. One of the nurses assisted me in putting on my loosely fitting jogging outfit and tennis shoes. Those were the clothes I was instructed to wear. Then a slim, attractive woman dressed in crisp white linen shorts arrived from the guest home. She helped me into the wheelchair and then into the Rolls Royce. I remained at The Hidden Garden for two days. The most unpleasant after-effects of the surgery was a day and a half of nausea due to the anesthesia. It prevented me from enjoying the spa cuisine and watching old movies as I had planned. I went home on Saturday. A close friend stayed with me for two days. Friends and relatives began phoning Saturday afternoon. Sunday night six of them came over. They were loaded down with a blender, two weeks supply of soft food (my jaws were sore and my ability to chew limited), and an enormous supply of good cheer. During the two weeks I was at home, I received between six and nine phone calls a day. Everyone, from my eleven year old niece to my eighty-six year old mother, was enthusiastic about what I had done. One of my friends commented, "Everyone I know would like to have done what you did but you are the only person I know who had the money and guts to do it." She added, "I think it takes more guts than money." I experienced an easy and uncomplicated recovery. At no time was I in any intense distress. I think the words weak, low level pain, and soreness best describe how I felt. The soreness was from the bruising under my eyes and the tissue tightening in my jaw. Five days after surgery I went out to lunch with a friend. Sore jaw or not I needed to eat something besides soft food. I ordered a cheese burger and french fries. It hurt to chew but it was worth it. From that time on I ate out almost every day. I began going shopping with friends and relatives and was driving the second week after surgery. During the two weeks I remained at home, I alternately rested and began taking short walks around the neighborhood. I tried to achieve a balance between obtaining sufficient rest and regaining my stamina. I wanted to be in adequate condition to deal with my patients and their problems when I returned to work.

People have inquired about my relatively quick and uncomplicated recovery. I think that several factors played a part. First of all I was in good physical condition. I am five feet four, weigh one hundred seventeen pounds, and don't have any physical illnesses. I jog three or four times a week, hike, swim, and exercise while watching the news. I don't smoke and rarely drink. Secondly, I feel better emotionally than I have at any time in my life. I love my work and enjoy my social life. Thirdly, I had a large (fifty in all), very positive support group. No one voiced anything negative about my having a facelift. Eleven of my friends and relatives instructed me to keep all the information on cosmetic surgery I had gathered since they would like to use it in the future. Additionally, most of the time I was aware that any discomfort I was undergoing was time limited. I also enjoy humor so I was able to view some aspects of my experience with humor, albeit black humor at times. Furthermore, I had planned a ski trip two months from the date of the surgery. I was looking forward to wearing the new ski outfits I had bought and again trying my hand at downhill racing.

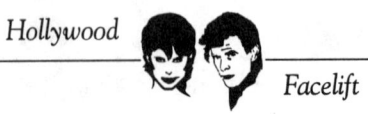

I returned to my practice two weeks following surgery. As luck would have it, the first patient I saw at six in the morning was a plastic surgeon. He was in analysis so typically would lie down on the couch. This hour he refrained from lying down on the couch, unsure I was well enough to deal with his problems. He did wonder if I thought my surgeon was more competent than he. The next day he entered the office, looked at me, said, "Well, you seem to be OK," and laid down on the couch. He proceeded to free associate about feeling abandoned by me just when he needed me most. Several days later I saw a seventeen year old girl, whom I had been seeing for four years. After initially inquiring about my well-being, giving her stamp of approval to my face, she proceeded to be critical of me for being so irresponsible. How could I have taken two weeks off from my patients for something as trivial as cosmetic surgery? Didn't I know that her parents were thinking of separating, she was getting a "D" in algebra, and had broken up with her boyfriend? Why wasn't I available to her when she needed me the most?

The following day I saw an eight year old girl, whom I had seen since she was three. When I entered the waiting room, she stared at my face and commented, "You look different, are you really Dr. Geller?" I tried to reassure her that I was Dr. Geller. Yet she kept asking, "Are you sure you are Dr. Geller?" Her mother quickly solved the problem by commenting, with a straight face, "Cynthia, that's Dr. Geller *fifteen years ago*." Cynthia's six year old sister added, "You don't have anymore wrinkles in your face, but *now* you have to do your hands."

My patients seemed to adjust well to my slightly altered appearance. I knew that my therapeutic approach had to be one which focused on the meaning my facelift had for them. And I could not sidestep their negative reactions. Nonetheless, I was surprised by the positive response of the mothers of young children. When I inquired about this, they, in essence, said the fact that my facelift turned out so well gave them hope. They knew that I had a grown daughter. They concluded if I could have gone through raising a child and at the end still be able to focus on myself, so could they. If needed, they too would have a facelift when they finished raising their children. I was a symbol to them that there was life after children.

Immediately after the surgery my relatives and friends were curious about how my face looked. Since I was not curious, this created some internal conflict. Furthermore, I found myself avoiding looking in the mirror. When I did, it was only for short time periods. Furthermore, I found it uncomfortable to carry on an extended conversation about my appearance. Focusing on my face was not enjoyable, even though people commented on how well it looked. What does one do when others are focusing on your face and the more they focus on it, the more anxious you become? Most of my life I seldom put much effort into my appearance. I regarded my face as quite ordinary. Now people were using words like attractive, pretty, and even beautiful. Entering professional, as well as social situations, where people have not seen me since my surgery is especially upsetting. Typically people remark on how well I look. They attribute my increased attractiveness to weight loss, a new hair style or being rested. Two months post-surgery I attended a Christmas party. A friend approached me and effusively remarked on how well I looked. In a bold voice she exclaimed, "You look terrific. What did you have done, a facelift?" I matter of factly replied, "Yes." She turned red, became flustered and questioned, "You did? I always say that to everyone who I think looks good. You are the only one who ever said 'yes'." I do not inform people that I have had a facelift unless they express bewilderment about my changed appearance. But I also don't hide it. I feel more comfortable when I am straightforward about it.

One of my unanticipated responses to the plastic surgery was that it significantly increased my sense of vulnerability. It also heightened my fear of bodily harm. Undoubtedly, this was due to the low level pain and bruising I initially experienced. As previously stated the surgery took five and a half hours and left me with over two hundred and fifty stitches in my scalp, face and neck. The physical trauma also caused some of my hair to fall out. As a result of my increased sense of vulnerability, I was watchful of people's rapid body movements. I became hypervigilant about doors being opened and closed too quickly. I also became fearful of other cars coming too close to mine when I was driving. I began worrying about germs and the possibility of infection. I found myself thinking, "What would happen if a suture site in my scalp became infected and then the infection spread to my brain, etc." Mental health workers usually regard people needing to use handkerchiefs to protect themselves from germs on door knobs as pathological. I now found myself thinking, "What is so pathological about that?" It seemed quite logical to me. This state of hypervulnerability and hypervigilance continued until two months after surgery. At that time I went on a five day ski trip, and I was able to ski four or five hours a day with no ill effects. Most importantly, the stitches across the crown of my head did not come loose. Although I know it was not logical, I had the visual image of me coming down a ski slope and the skin in my forehead coming undone. I went on two more ski trips after the first, respectively three and four months post-surgery. The third trip found my fear and caution so greatly reduced, that I was able to take part in a NASTAR downhill race. I was beginning to place my surgical procedure into the frame of reference of being part of a routine course of events. That was until my surgeon made a comment during one of my monthly examinations. We were discussing the possibility of my having a chemical peel to reduce the fine lines around my eyes. In this procedure, a chemical is applied to the face to remove the skin's most wrinkled top layers. It is performed under local anesthesia and does produce some redness and swelling. During this conversation, the surgeon looked me squarely in the eye and said, "Shirley, I want to tell you, you really have guts and courage to go through all of this." I thought to myself, "Here I have been regarding all of this, nausea from anesthesia, low level pain, physical weakness and hair loss, as normal and *now* you tell me I have guts and courage to go through all of this. Why didn't you tell me this when we began?" As the conversation progressed my surgeon divulged that three years ago he had had his eyelids done and almost canceled out the night before. Anxiety almost got the better of him.

Although not completely conscious on my part, I think some of my motivation for having a facelift was to turn back the clock. Nevertheless, I was unprepared for what it would mean to experience the Rip Van Winkle effect in reverse. My first encounter with people responding to me as if I was ten to fifteen years younger occurred a month after surgery. I went to the local hardware store to buy a barbecue spit, volcanic rock, and barbecue utensils for a dinner I was having at my house. The cashier took my check and asked for my driver's license for identification. After noting my date of birth on the license, she informed me I qualified for the senior citizen discount. The store gave ten percent off to customers fifty-five and over. She rang up my items and placed my check in the cash register. Then, for the first time during our transaction, she looked up at me. She gazed at my face, looked at my date of birth on the driver's license and angrily declared, "Say, you're not fifty-five, you don't qualify for our senior citizen discount." I leaned over the counter and in a softer tone informed her I had just had a facelift. As a result, I looked younger than I was. With that she removed her glasses and showed me her eyelids. She inquired as to how I thought she would look if the fatty deposits were removed? She asked for the name of my surgeon. And she gave me my discount.

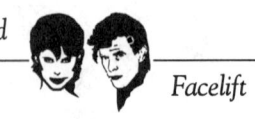

Since I have had my facelift, I notice that people are spontaneously talking to me with greater frequency and for longer periods of time. Additionally, younger individuals are stopping to carry on casual conversations.

On the last ski club trip I found myself engaged in conversation with a thirty-eight year old man. He asked to buy me a drink, began questioning me as to what plays and movies I preferred. He then asked what type of men I liked to date. There was something vaguely familiar about this conversation. After a few minutes I realized I was in a time warp. I had experienced similar types of conversations, but I had experienced them twenty-some years ago. Outwardly I continued talking. Inwardly I wondered what was I going to do with this situation. I felt an urge to inform this verbal, smiling man that I was not as young as I looked.

During the same evening, I was speaking to a woman about my twenty-one year old daughter. She commented that it was nice my daughter and I could "grow up together." I didn't comprehend what she was implying. When questioned her about her comment she said, "You are probably around thirty-eight or thirty-nine, or at the most in your early forties so you and your daughter grew up together." I declared I was fifty-five. She looked shocked and replied, "Oh, come on, you're putting me on." It was then I revealed to her I had recently had a facelift.

A week ago I ran into a social worker, whom I hadn't seen in thirteen years. His hair was grey and his face wrinkled and sagging. We used to work together at the same child guidance clinic. Martin looked at my face, shook his head in disbelief and said, "Shirley, you are the same. You haven't changed a bit since the last time I saw you." I impulsively replied, "Martin, I have changed. The only reason I look like I haven't changed is because I recently had a facelift."

Originally I wanted a facelift so that my face would be more congruent with my psyche. I am now having experiences in which my face is incongruent with my chronological age. This I find quite unnerving. Five months have passed since my surgery. Having a facelift so far has certainly been a series of adventures, and I am not sure what the future will hold.

Every now and then I think back on how this all started. "Dr. Geller, you have more wrinks."

Nola's Note: "A Wrinkle In Time" is taken from the children's book by the same title.

What's "Hot" In Beverly Hills

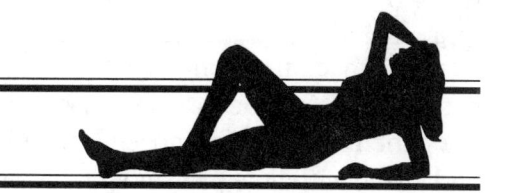

Goodbye To A Shiny Head!

Dr. Richard Fleming and Dr. Toby Mayer, both full plastic surgeons, are co-directors of The Beverly Hills Institute of Aesthetic & Reconstructive Surgery[12] in Beverly Hills. They are internationally known for their hair replacement technique known as the "Fleming/Mayer Flap." The surgeon takes large sections of hair bearing scalp and rotates them from the sides and back to bald areas. (Several flaps may be necessary.) Because the hair is never totally separated from its blood supply, there is no temporary hair loss. The hair density is uniform and as thick as the hair on the sides of the head. This allows for easy and varied hair styling. Fleming/Mayer Flap patients can comb their hair straight back or part it anywhere. They can swim, play tennis or engage in any type of sport without worrying about their appearance. Coverage is *immediate!*

Results: Incredible!

A Baby's Skin!

Cristina Carlino skin care products and treatments sold under the name BIOMEDIC Clinical Care[13] has carefully developed facial peels. Conservatively evaluating the patient's skin type, the skin care analyst designs a peel solution to meet your individual needs. Unlike the strong Phenol or Chemical Peel, she designs a light to medium strength acid solution (resorcinol, salicylic, lactic and/or glycolic acid) according to skin color, skin type, skin age, skin tone and skin texture . . . your skin.

Cristina has a "Micro Peel." It takes twenty to thirty minutes—a lunch hour peel—and in seven days your skin is clean, clear, healthy and glowingly young and looks well-scrubbed for months! The way the light peel works is simple: The caustic substances burns the skin like a sunburn. On the fourth day, a thin layer of tanned skin just peels off. The process makes the complexion smoother and younger looking! It can be repeated as needed, and can be used on the neck and hands.

Results in seven days: Incredible!

Monday A.M. Facelift—Wednesday P.M. Dinner Party Date!

Glue made from one's own plasma has been successfully used by John E. Williams, M.D.,[14] located at Museum Square on Wilshire Boulevard. A week in advance, a pint of blood is taken from the patient and the fibrinogen isolated and frozen. At the time of surgery, the fibrinogen is thawed and mixed with an equal amount of commercially-prepared thrombin. This glue type mixture is used during surgery, accelerating coagulation while adhering to wounds. This fibrin network sets up quickly and has strong adhesive properties.

Its use in a facelift minimizes complications. We have definitely seen less bruising and less swelling here at The Hidden Garden. Although used in Europe, fibrin glue made from the patient's own blood is beginning to be more widely used here.

Results: Saves one to two weeks in healing time, important if you have a hot date!

Hot Lips!

For those desperate for permanent puffy lips, this may be the answer! Your body does not fully reject your own body's fat. Michael Churukian, M.D.,[15] in Beverly Hills, has effectively and easily injected fat from the low abdomen into the lip area creating fuller more youthful lips. Although the long term retention is 10-20% for each injection, after several injections over a period of twelve to eighteen months a build up of fat can occur. Depending on your body's rate of absorption, this could lead to "permanent" puffy lips. Call for info.

Results: So far—Incredible! Worth checking out!

Peaches And Cream Complexions!

For those of us that have developed that "red face" look due to the small red capillaries under our thin, translucent skin, especially around the nose and cheek areas—Good news! Adrianna Scheibner, M.D.,[16] on Bedford Drive is a master perfectionist with her fine laser beam. Gently and quickly she will treat those tiny red capillaries and believe me, you will have a wonderful new complexion.

Results: Healing time is two weeks to up to a month...and you look awful. *But it is well worth it!*

Wake Up To Looking Your Best!

Permanent cosmetic makeup, or cosmetic tattooing, is a permanent "never have to do again" deposit of color into the dermis. Derma Pigmentation developed by Sheila May,[17] a medical tatoo artist, can be a lifesaver for those who are allergic to eye cosmetics, wear contacts or for those who are finding it harder to apply their make-up. Various procedures include: eyebrows, lip liner, and eye liner for both upper and lower eyes. The results are subtle and natural. It is painless and can be applied as lightly or as heavily as you desire. Color choices are also available. It is such a great procedure that you may want to add a little beauty mark or go wild with a real *tattoo!*

Sheila can make surgical scars disappear. She tattoos the scar to match your natural skin color. Perfect for facial scars, hairline scars or even breast scars. It is quick and painless.

Result: Immediate.

"Hot . . . . . Hot": Skin Resurfacing

Laser technology is revolutionizing the field of plastic surgery. Just a few years ago, lasers were rarely used by plastic surgeons. Today, lasers are used for purposes ranging from resurfacing of the skin to tattoo removal. This technique of facial skin resurfacing uses the carbon dioxide (CO2) laser, a process also known as **laserbrasion**. Frank H. Ryan, M.D.[18] specializing in this new technique will send you more information.

Result: Excellent.

What's Really "Hot"

A new method of performing browlifts (or forehead lifts) is now being performed. The "Endoscopic Browlift" borrows technology used by the orthopedic surgeon in performing arthroscopic surgery. Several small (one inch) incisions are made in the scalp and specially designed instruments are placed beneath the forehead. The surgeon watches the instruments on a video monitor and is able to remove the muscles that cause the frown lines between the eyebrows. He also is able to elevate the eyebrow to a more youthful, rested-appearing position. Be sure to go to a surgeon well experienced in this technique. An excellent source for this new technique is Robert W. Hutcherson[19], M.D., Co-Director of the Endoscopic Facial Surgery Program at U.C.L.A.

Result: Excellent.

It's All In The Timing

Doctors are believing that the healing process is faster and the results better for women before menopause.

As a woman's body ages, a substance called estrogen begins to become just as important as her cholesterol count. The lack of estrogen seems to hasten the aging process. With aging, the cell renewal process slows, healing takes longer. As our skin produces less collagen, the skin loses its natural bounce and snug fit. The more estrogen, the more collagen, the better the result and the longer the result. Plastic surgeons and gynecologists are agreeing that pre-menopausal women are better candidates for a facelift. Average age of a Hollywood Facelift is forty-five.

Result: Always looking good.

> **Plastic surgery will not stop "Mother Nature" but regardless of age, you will always look better for the rest of your life!**

The New You!

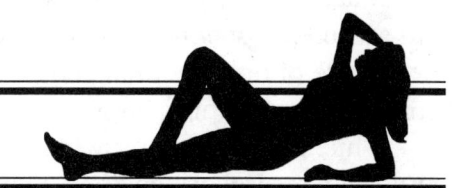

If we were to ask each man and each woman who has stayed at The Hidden Garden exactly what made them decide to have a facelift, many would have one thing in common, it happened at a low time in their lives. A time when they were feeling a "less worth" about themselves. Perhaps at a time when there was a re-evaluation or breakup of a personal relationship, a realization that the years have physically caught up with them or perhaps at a time of a need for change.

Many cosmetic surgery patients go into surgery with a low or poor self-esteem but who emerge after their surgery with a renewed excitement, a renewal energy, a new feeling of competence, a new love for life. They gain a sense of control over their life rather than being a victim of events.

Out of desperation after a divorce, one may choose to have a facelift to look younger to attract a new male companion. What usually happens is the fact that one looks so good (the loss of ten years) that one no longer is desperate, one feels great and starts to enjoy being single. This person's new inner, more self-confident self shines through and a new personality develops. This individual becomes more attractive and new friendships are created. The results are even better than expected. You have a new more attractive and happier you.

Cosmetic surgery cannot give you personal security but it can help you attain a higher level of self-esteem. Many times we can feel temporarily "low" or hopeless, overwhelmed and through a cosmetic procedure, a procedure we have wanted to do, for ourselves, we have the strength to start moving ahead again.

Life becomes a challenge again.

Most cosmetic surgery patients do it for themselves. They want to look as "good as they feel." That seems to be the strong motivation behind the decision to have a facelift. However, plastic surgery does affect your self-esteem. Even if you did not intend it to do so, it will. People will react to you differently. They will make comments, "How young you look!" "How good your skin looks." These comments will reinforce your new look and encourage you to put on the finishing touches. To lose a few pounds, change your hair color, feel more comfortable in a different style dress, or perhaps not have to hide behind pounds of jewelry.

This "feeling good about oneself" can trigger a renewed energy with one's career, even result in higher achievements. But it is wrong to expect that the "new look" will change one's total personalty, that you will be far more successful or have more pleasant sexual encounters. That would be a big mistake.

When we feel good about ourselves, we talk with ease, we are more friendly and spontaneous. An attitude of openness and curiosity about new ideas, an excitement for new experiences and a new sense of humor draws people to you. Not being at war with oneself, a quiet inner harmony comes through. This quality is very attractive.

While we do not know what actually influences self-esteem, whether the factors are biological or developmental, we do know that there are specific practices that can raise or lower it. And the results of a facelift, breast augmentation (or reduction), a tummy tuck or liposuction can manifest itself in the way we walk, talk, even in our expressions of affection.

When we look good, we feel good and no longer need to hide behind jewelry, clothes, hair or excessive body fat. We are more relaxed and happier. We enjoy being who we are.

Not only has the cosmetic surgery procedure taken years off your looks but can save on expensive shopping trips for new clothes, cosmetics, etc., to satisfy a need and it can save on additional therapy sessions because you have become a more healthy, independent person. Cosmetic surgery can result in a psychological victory.

We refer to "facelifts" as having a major effect on one's life. But other surgeries also are equally as effective. Breast implants are most popular with women in their forties after having several children. Sagging breasts are such a "turn-off" to husbands and a disappointment to the woman. Men are not crazy (contrary to the "Playboy" image) about huge breasts, but they are not happy with sagging breasts, either. The new saline implants placed under the muscle are safe and feel natural and look natural. It is not necessary to go to a "bigger" cup size. A minor breast reduction can be performed at the same time. In fact, breast reductions amongst young women are happening by the thousands throughout the United States. No longer are young girls going through the embarrassments and harassments that very large breasts can cause.

While women are having their sagging breasts augmented, they are having the extra fat removed from their waistlines, a new figure all at once. Now wouldn't that bring new life to a marriage!

Who you are includes how you look, which in turn gives us an image of who you are. It is important to focus on our total whole life, how we want to live our life and "how we look" is an aspect of our life.

"In our getting culture, physical appearance has a big impact on how we're perceived, which in turn often influences what and how much we're able and unable to get—dates, attention in the shoe store, jobs, and a whole lot more besides. If we appear to be too fat or too old, disabled or disfigured, or if we don't have the right clothes or the right kind of nose, we're more likely to get turned down, ignored or dismissed than those who've got "good looks." Which isn't to say that good-looking people don't also have to deal with other people's competitiveness, which can be expressed in ways that are hurtful and even hostile. But it is a fact of life in our culture that appearances, while they aren't everything, mean a lot."

> "Millions of women chose to 'make themselves up' for fun, to show their style ... in the spirit of giving. Their "fashion statement" is "I'm doing this not because I have to, but because I want to."[20]

What You Can Do To Hide An Old Look

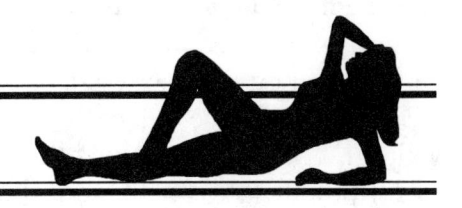

Plastic surgery is not for everyone. This book is written to help you make that decision. Once you know your options, what is available, the risks and results, and the costs, you can proceed with your life.

The beauty magazines are filled with suggestions for looking good without plastic surgery. However, they are in the business of *selling* cosmetics, clothes, etc. The following ten celebrity beauty rules for an ANTI-AGE LOOK are within reach and pocketbook of everyone.

Anti-Aging Rule #1: MAKE DO WITH LESS MAKEUP.

Clean, glowing skin with the "suggestion" of lip color, eye liner and blush is very youthful. Yet we insist on layers and layers of foundation to hide the flaws. The way to good skin is to have an A.M. and P.M. cleaning regimen. The daily mild peels will definitely help in this area, as well as the weekly and monthly deeper treatments. Facial scrubs and products with alpha hydroxy acid are exfoliants which draw fluid into the area, leaving skin smoother and brighter. Permanent makeup is an excellent investment at this time.

Anti-Aging Rule #2: LOCK THE JEWELRY BOX.

Selecting one fine piece of jewelry draws attention to the piece — a conversation item. Overloading our body with every piece we own is not only distasteful but unattractive. Is it that we want to show off our jewelry collection all at once? Being selective or choosing only one piece of a set is not only more attractive, it takes years off your look. How many younger women load themselves down? Think simplicity when it comes to selecting our accessories. A hat, hair pin, glasses, earrings, necklace, bracelet, watch, belt, pin, gloves, buttons, and fancy shoes worn all at one time will create a comic look. Not a look that's particularly attractive. Only a few of us can wear such a look successfully. Think about it!

Anti-Aging Rule #3: HEALTHY HAIR.

The hair on your head frames your face. Why do all sixty year olds have the same hair cut and style? You need to get out of that rut! Hairstyle is a dead giveaway to your age. Pick a style ten years younger, a hair color with highlights. Avoid a one colored hair style and avoid hair spray. It's natural for your locks to be soft and a little "relaxed." This "unset" look will actually take less time and less visits to the hairdresser. Hair should be "perky," not too long, not to serious. Don't be afraid to go a little "wild"!!

Anti-Aging Rule #4: CHOOSE YOUR EYEGLASS FRAMES CAREFULLY.

After fifty, glasses are a must. But why is it we never consider the frames as an important statement of our image? We purchase frames like chunks of costume jewelry, great for one occasion, out of place for everything else, yet we wear our glasses very day. Pick a look: school girl, Granny, office girl, 40's single — but be true to that look. Or have several pair of glasses, like any accessory. *AND* carefully select your glasses along with the jewelry that you are wearing. A dead giveaway is the woman in eyeglasses overloaded with huge dangling ear and neck jewels. Better yet: get contact lenses.

Anti-Aging Rule #5: PEARLY WHITE TEETH AGAIN.

Our teeth become stained with years of coffee and tea drinking, smoking and even by some antibiotics. Teeth whitening is an inexpensive procedure. This bleaching process requires only two to four office visits and brightens tooth enamel without damaging healthy teeth. Teeth that have been discolored with age will become light again very easily. This whitening effect will last for several years and may easily be repeated. The cost is $200-$600 and is a wonderful investment.

Anti-Aging Rule #6: PERFECT YOUR SMILE.

Another worthwhile investment is in your smile. The vertical lines forming around the lips are a dead giveaway to our age. Several treatments, used continuously, have proven successful and a noticeable change will be seen. Use an exfoliant to remove dead surface cells, this forces new cells to surface. Products with alpha hydroxy acids (at least 12%), used daily, can make this lip area smoother and fine lines less noticeable, or try fat injections.

Anti-Aging Rule #7: EAT WELL FOR A HEALTHY GLOW.

Our bodies absorb less proteins and nutrients and it actually takes more vitamins and minerals for us to function as we get older. Our bodies do not fully absorb the vitamins and minerals as it did ten years earlier. Perhaps we need to re-evaluate our diets, drink less alcohol, eat less white bread, pasta, and pastry, less sugar and salt, but eat more low fat protein, fruits and vegetables, and add vitamin and mineral supplements as needed.

As we get older, we prepare meals that are "easy," not necessarily as nutritious as they could be. The object as we get older is to not eat more calories, but to actually eat less calories but more nutrient rich calories. Just as we should be eating to preserve our health, we are not. It is a medical fact that good nutrition plays an important part in the aging process. Plan meals. Enjoy the dining experience. Make it special.

Make grocery shopping fun. Many towns have encouraged local growers to set up the weekly "Open Markets." It is not only fun to shop, but the produce is fresher and usually "vine ripe," making it more nutritious.

The **Hollywood Facelift Diet** suggestions can help you plan your meals.

Anti-Aging Rule #8: GET OFF THE COUCH

Thanks to the many new video tapes and T.V. programs, we are exposed to exercising on all levels. How you walk, how you move, how you carry yourself all give your age away.

Pick a sport. No one says you have to be good at it. Just do it regularly.

Many people hate the gym, thirty to forty minutes once a week is all they can stand. But if they combine that gym visit with a weekly walk on the beach, an exercise/yoga class, a cowboy "two stepping" class, "swing" class, or even an Arthur Murray "ballroom" dance class and one forty-five minute home video "stretching" workout, you have with very little effort and no pain increased your circulation, your flexibility, your metabolism, your spirits and have had fun doing it.

Anti-Aging Rule #9: TIMELESS DRESSING.

New mini skirts may not be for you. And I don't want to see my eighty year old mother in Levis. But there is something "timeless" about a white linen suit or a pair of khaki twill pants and tweed jacket with classic leather loafers. Who can guess your age? In fact, they won't even think of you and age, they will place you in an age bracket, and keeping you there for the next ten years. A newly fifty-five year old woman didn't mind the gossip at the Christmas party when her friends and guests couldn't put their finger on her real age, "She must be forty-five, or is it fifty?" yet they had known her for years. She quietly takes ten years off her daughter's age just to complete the picture. People are always adding up years in their head, "If her daughter is twenty, she must be forty-five." She smiles as she walks gracefully off in her "timeless" black dress which she wears each year to this special event.

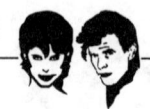

Anti-Aging Rule #10: AGE IS AN ATTITUDE.

People who are excited about life, who continue to learn new things, who look for the positive in their lives, not only look younger, feel younger, they are younger. Age is an attitude.

Getting out of the house and into a bridge class or yoga group, a writing class, a film screening discussion group ... or just a walk to the library is the first step. And the first step is always the hardest. There are many people out there just starting a new venture at sixty-five. The retired gentleman who took up tennis and plays two hours a day every day is still playing at eighty-five; the lady who just got a job at a major department store, or the gentleman who turned his garage hobby into a small business and seven years later, sold his business for over a million dollars, and is still working as their consultant at the age of seventy-two.

Age is an attitude.

The Hollywood Facelift

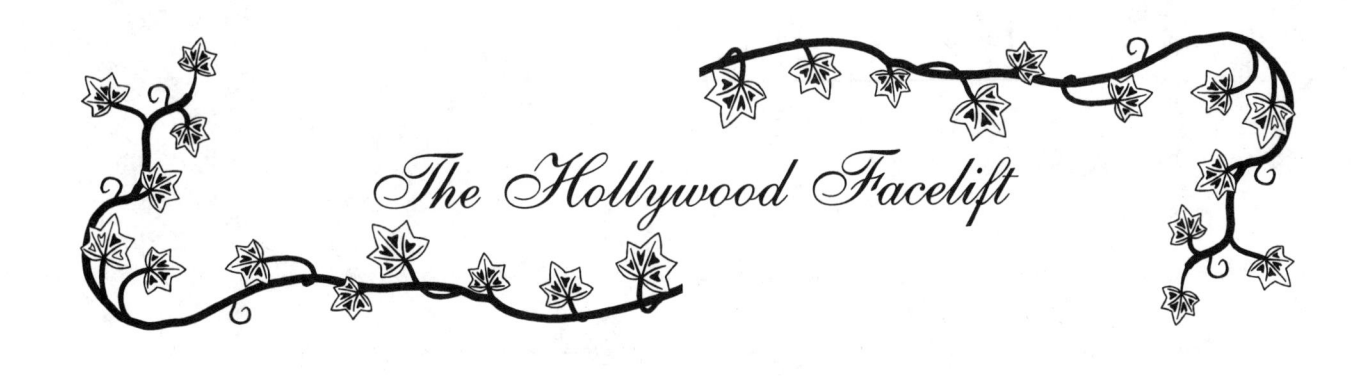

The Lighter Side

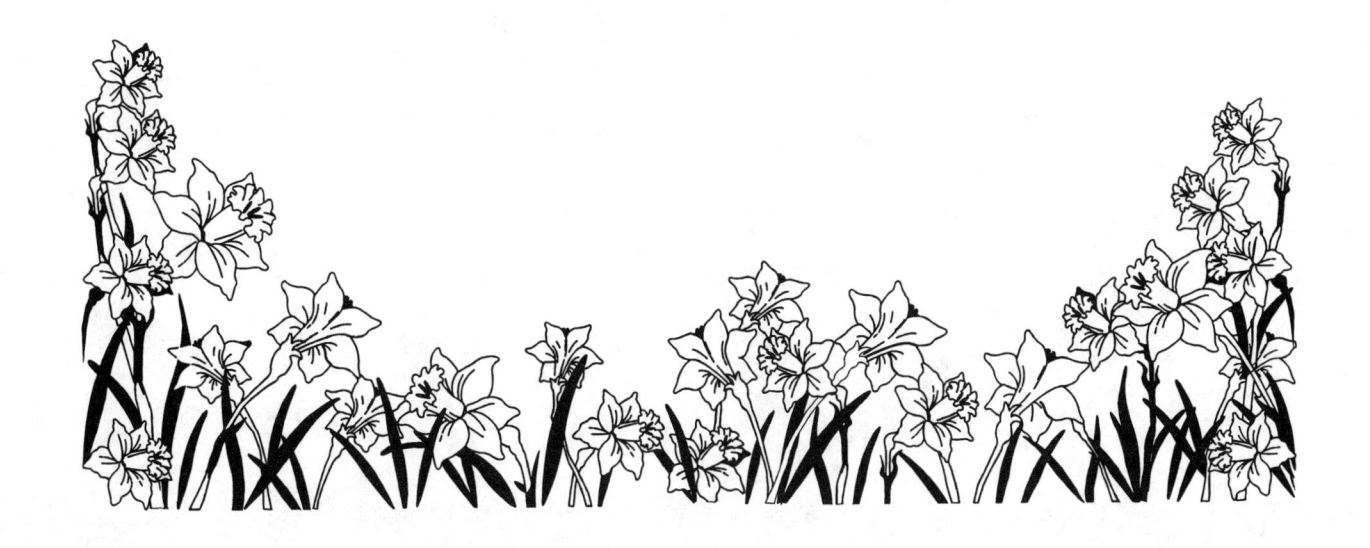

The Lighter Side

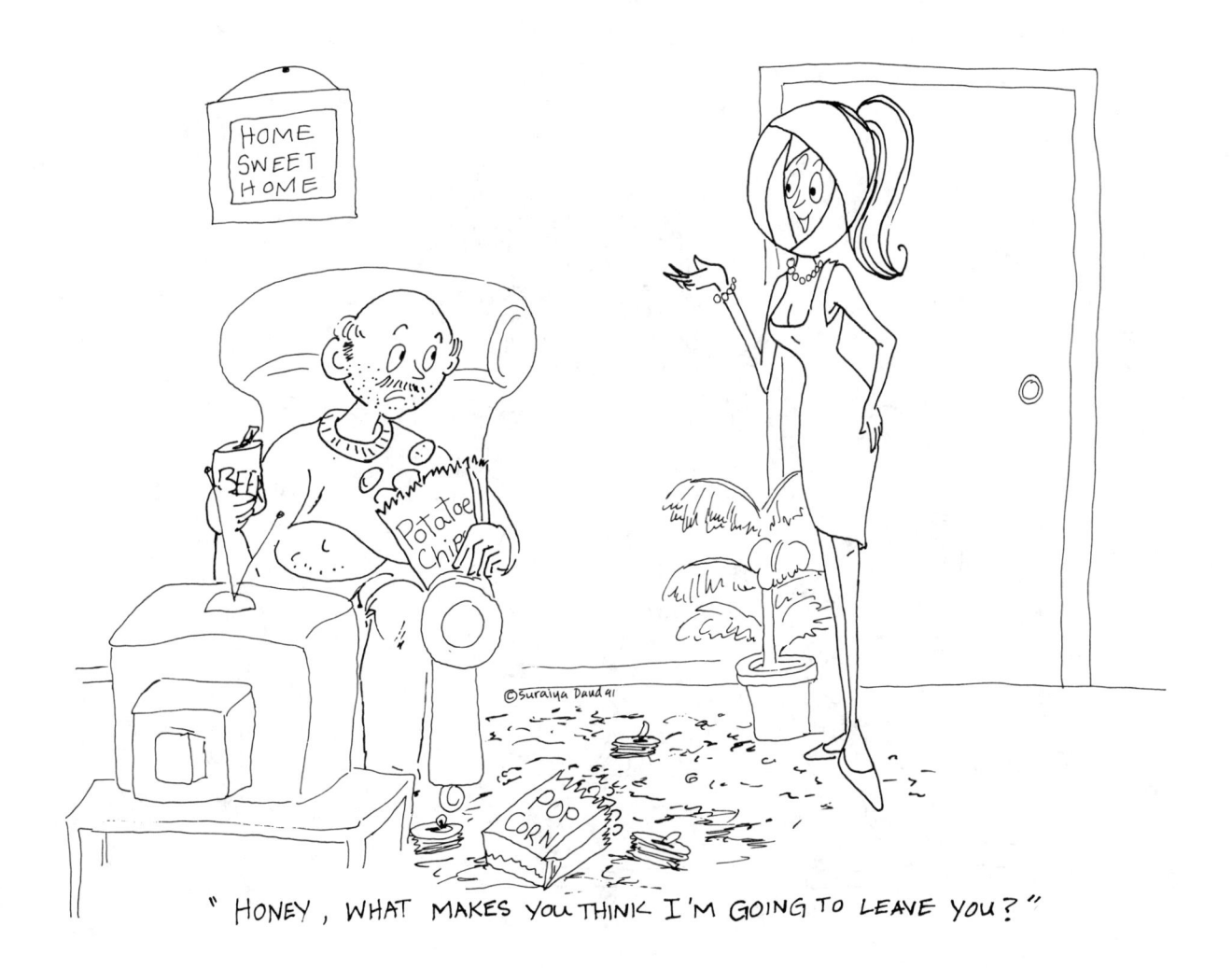

"HONEY, WHAT MAKES YOU THINK I'M GOING TO LEAVE YOU?"

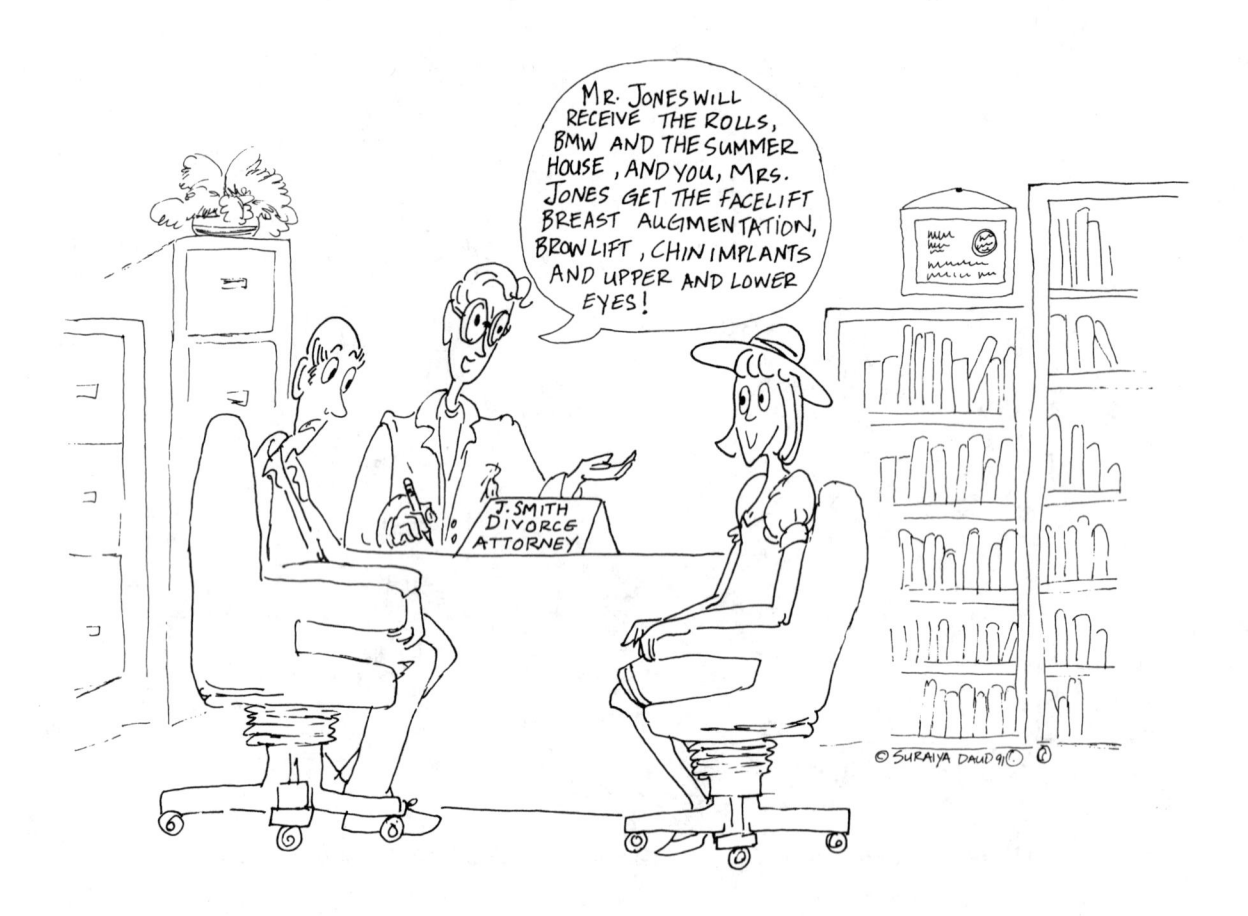

The Hollywood Facelift

The Lighter Side

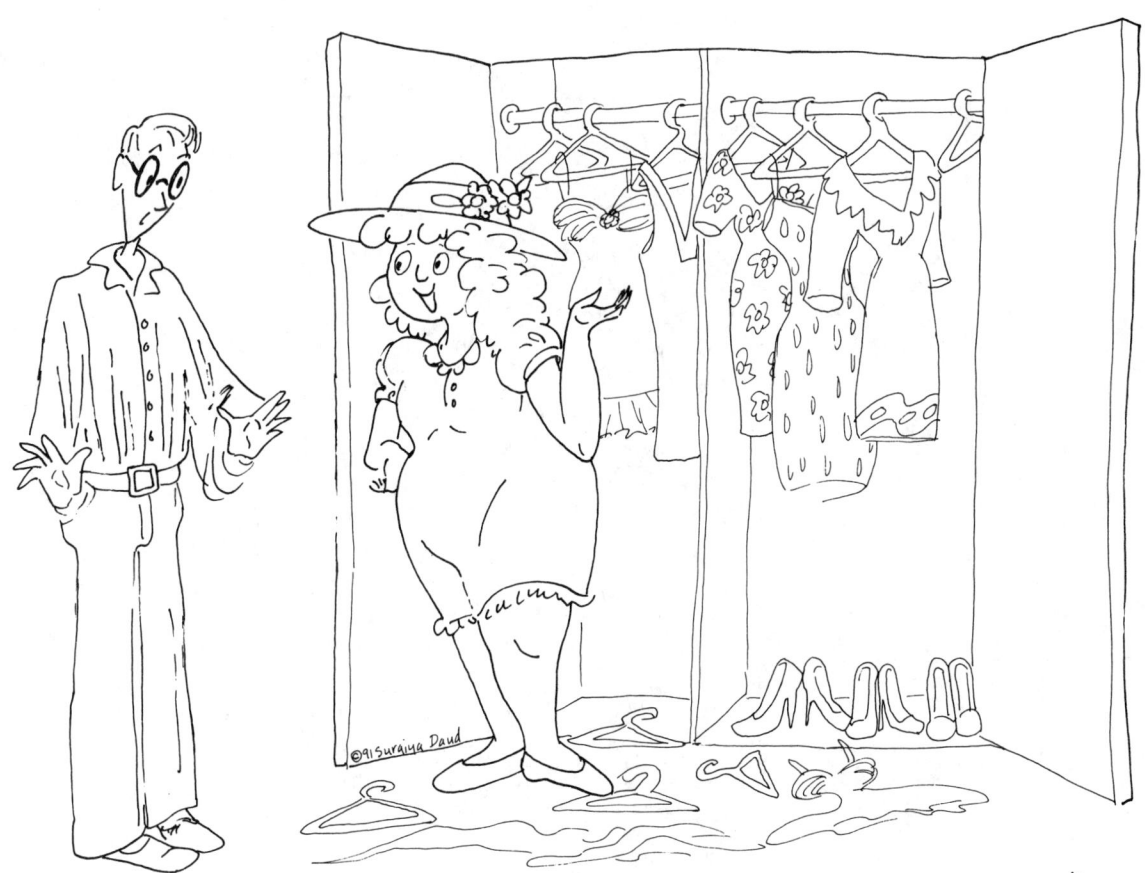

"HONEY, LIPO IS CHEAPER THAN A NEW WARDROBE."

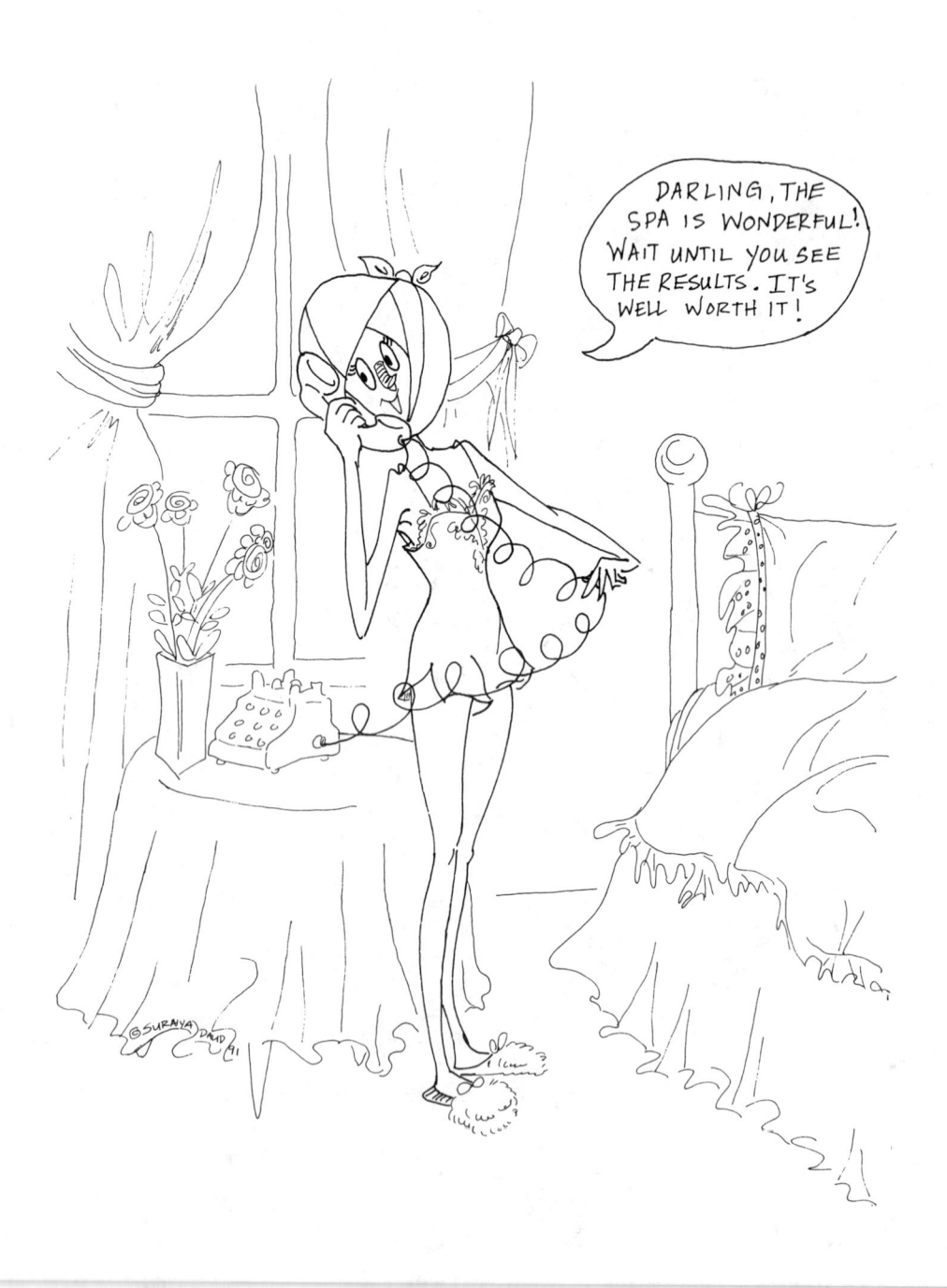

The Hollywood Facelift

The Lighter Side

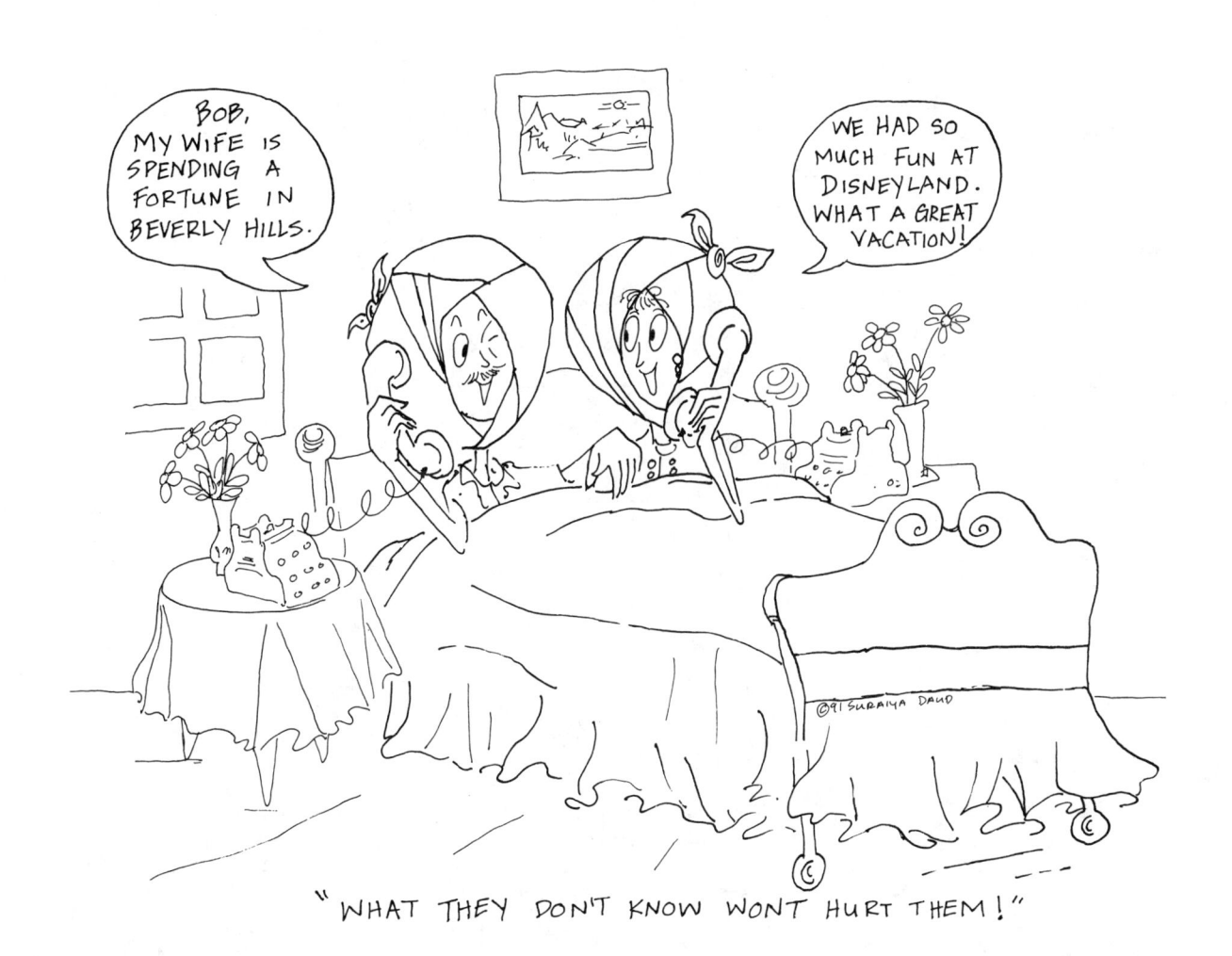

The Hollywood Facelift

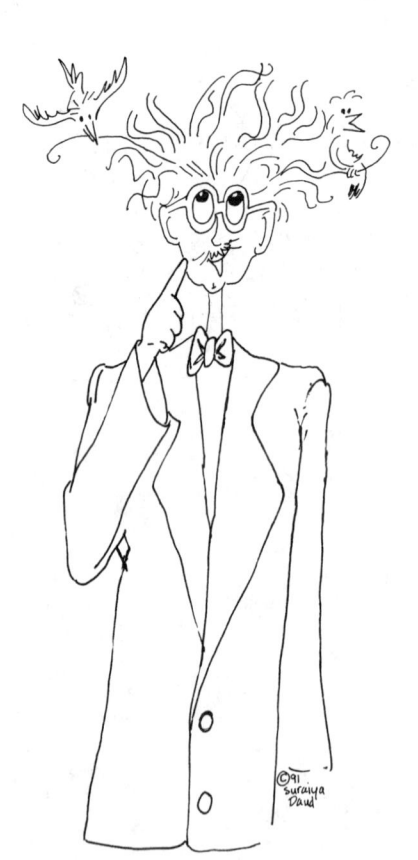

"One too many!"

The Hollywood Facelift Diet

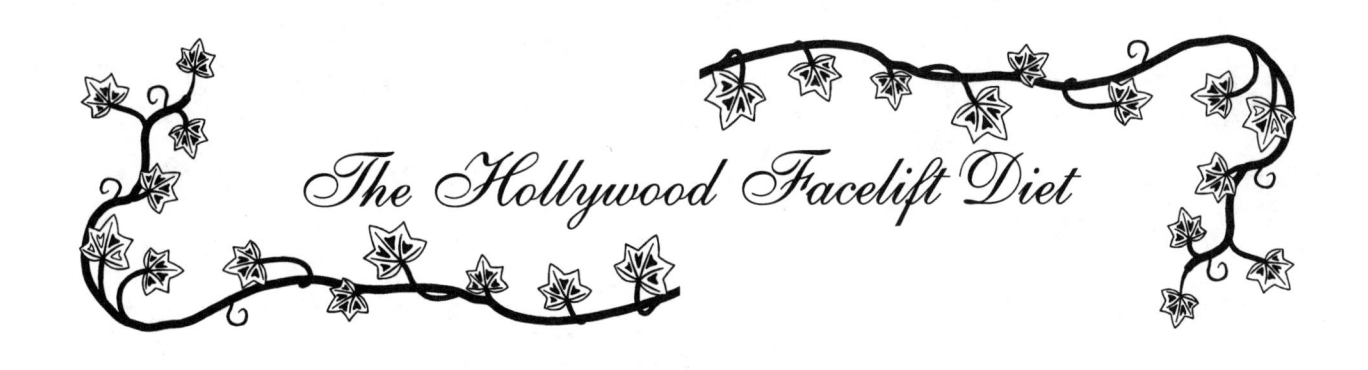

Part 2

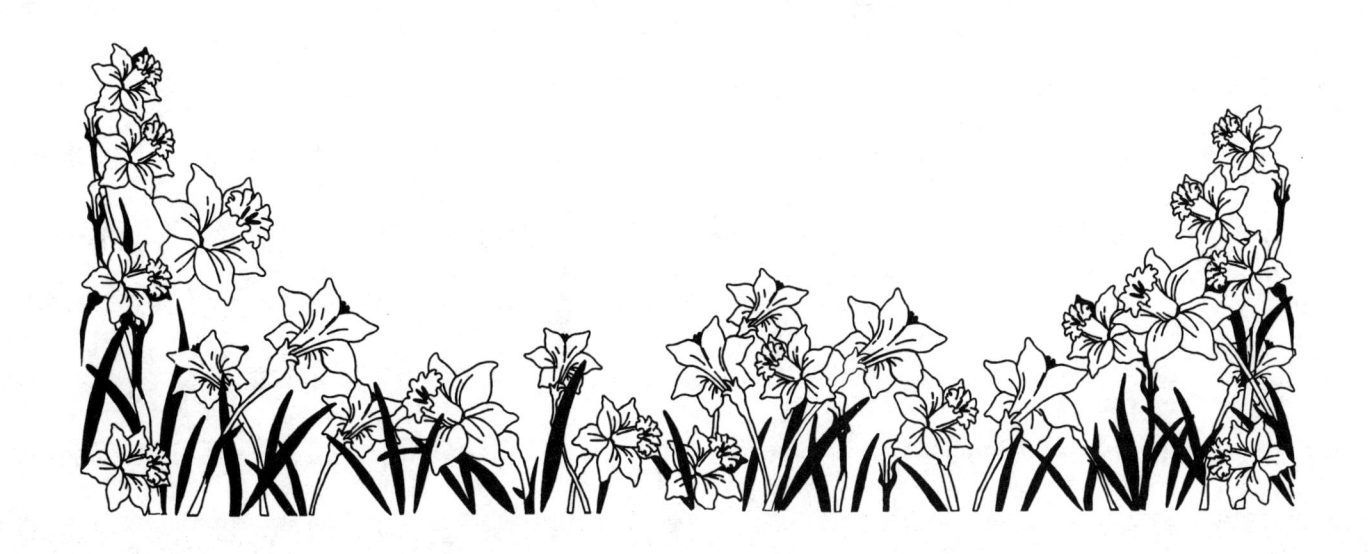

Introduction

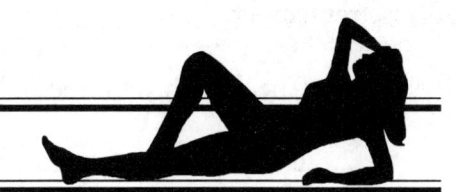

You do not need a facelift to benefit from this diet!! Today, our lifestyles are different. We drink more, we eat out more, we go on food rages—Chinese, Thai, Cajun, pizza, pasta. We are told as we get older that our metabolism changes and we gain about one pound per year without eating anything more. So, at forty-five we are 10 pounds heavier than we were at thirty-five, eating the exact same foods.

Your new face may encourage you to change your eating habits, especially if you need to lose a few pounds. Fortunately we are learning more about foods and exercise and **The Hollywood Facelift Diet** reflects this knowledge. It is well-balanced, delicious and very easy to prepare. The daily menus are a guide for surgery patients and in that respect, it's very important to follow them carefully.

The Hollywood Facelift Diet is specifically designed to be low in fats, salt and sugar, and it does not use preservatives or artificial coloring. It is high in fiber, iron and potassium.

The goal is to have a nutritious, well-balanced diet during the post-operative period as well as to enjoy delicious meals. We encourage Tea Time to include fresh fruits or fruit breads. One needs energy at this time of day.

Many guests have lost weight on this diet yet have not felt deprived. Our guests continue with our diet program at home after their three to four day stay at The Hidden Garden. They cannot believe that after eating all the foods that we serve, they have not gained weight. The daily food schedule, according to them, is a big help, especially the first ten days when they have a "finicky" appetite and cannot chew. Liposuction and breast surgery guests can follow **The Hollywood Facelift Diet**, but because they can chew they can substitute foods of equal nutritional value. During days #1-#20 for face surgeries guests, the important factor is the *texture* of the foods. For example, toast is too hard to chew, but certain types of muffins can be easily broken and crumbled. String beans are too fibrous and chicken must be finely-chopped. Guests allergic to certain foods or milk products are encouraged to use substitutes of equal amounts and nutritional value.

Because you need calories for healing, doctors do not want you on a "strict" diet. **The Hollywood Facelift Diet** has the perfect balance.

You will not only encourage optimum healing but you will feel good and look incredible from head to toe!

As a weight reduction diet, breakfasts, lunches and dinners can be interchanged but you must omit listed evening snack or substitute a fruit or sorbet. For a more rapid weight loss omit all pies, muffins, cookies, cakes and dessert breads. However, one day each week, choose a desert and enjoy it!

Please remember:

1. Check with your doctor before going on any diet!

2. Do not lose weight too quickly after your facelift or you will have facial contours that might be very unpleasant.

3. Do not gain weight either, you could encourage the scars to stretch and of course void your lift totally.

4. Do not lose weight *before* the surgery unless you do so at least five to six months in advance and remain at that weight for the two to three month period before your facelift.

5. Do change your eating style. Chances are that if you lose five to ten pounds, one to two months before surgery, you will gain some or all of it back. It takes time to establish a new "life style."

Diet Tricks:

1. Drink water throughout the day. Aim for eight full glasses.

Result: Stomach feels full.

2. Graze. Eat small nutritious snacks throughout the day. Have healthy mid-morning snacks and don't forget afternoon tea time. Avoid large meals, they stimulate the body to produce more insulin.

Result: Blood sugar levels remain more stable and the urge to eat is reduced.

3. Eat more soup.

Result: Soups are more filling with less calories.

4. Eat foods high in complex carbohydrates. The metabolic rate goes up.

Result: You feel satisfied sooner.

5. Eat slowly and chew food thoroughly.

Result: Eating slower means eating less food.

6. Substitute "fat free" whenever possible.

The Hollywood Facelift Diet

WEEK ONE - DAY # 1

Arrival Time:	Wild Strawberry Jello Slices of Banana Tea Biscuits
Dinner:	Apple Juice The Hidden Garden Homemade Chicken Soup* Mashed Potatoes Pureed Banana Squash Soft Crackers Mango Puree
Evening Snack:	Frozen Lemon Sorbet with Mint Leaf
Midnight Snack:	Strawberry-Banana Milkshake*, or Diane's Fruit Smoothie*, or Glass of Warm Milk

Nola's Note: It's hard to sleep the first night and a midnight snack is relaxing.

*See the Table of Contents for the recipe page numbers

WEEK ONE - DAY # 2

Breakfast:	Cream of Wheat, Sprinkles of Brown Sugar
	Scones w/Honey & Jam
	Finely Chopped Fresh Fruit Salad: Grapes, Strawberries, Melons, Stewed Prunes, Cantaloupe
	Non-fat Yogurt w/Drops of Honey
	Pineapple Juice
	Decaf Coffee
Mid-morning:	Zesty Kiwi, Banana Slices & Strawberries
Lunch:	Country Inn Potato Leek Soup* & Soft Crackers
	Chilled Pureed Mango
Tea Time:	Blueberry Milkshake* in a Chilled Parfait
Dinner:	Fresh Tomato Mushroom Bisque*
	Soft Crackers
	Scoop of "Real" Italian Country Style Polenta*
	Pear Juice
Evening Snack:	Chilled Raspberry Sorbet & a Soft Cookie

Nola's Note: Yogurt is served daily to avoid the possibilities of yeast infections due to antibiotics.

The Hollywood Facelift Diet

WEEK ONE - DAY # 3

Breakfast:	Egg whites scrambled w/white pepper
	Croissant/Fruit Preserve
	Non-fat Yogurt w/drops of honey
	Poached Pear*
	Mango Juice
	Decaf Coffee
Mid-morning:	Bowl of Stewed Prunes
Lunch:	Spinach & Mushroom Quiche
	Slivers of Steamed Carrots
	Wheat Roll
	Pineapple Juice or Apple Juice
Tea Time:	Strawberry-Banana Milkshake* w/extra berries
Dinner:	The Hidden Garden Homemade Manicotti* w/freshly chopped tomato & herb sauce
	Baked Scallopini Squash* brushed w/olive oil & dill
Evening Snack:	Scoop of Frozen Blueberry Yogurt

WEEK ONE - DAY # 4

Breakfast:	Old-Fashioned Quaker Oats or Oat Bran Blueberry Muffin & Jam Thin Slices of fresh Kiwi, Bananas, Melon Non-fat Yogurt w/Honey drops Mango Juice Decaf Coffee
Mid-morning:	Natural Cran/Apple Sauce served warm or cold w/Custard Sauce*
Lunch:	The Hidden Garden Homemade Carrot Soup* w/Sprig of Parsley Mint Cucumber Salad* Wheat Crackers
Tea Time:	Poached Pear* serve w/Cinnamon Stick Herb Tea

Dinner:	Broiled Chilean Sea Bass* served
	   w/Fresh Tomato-Basil Salad
	Baked Yam
	Steamed Fresh Chopped Spinach
	   w/drops of Olive Oil

Evening Snack:	Vanilla Non-fat Ice Cream w/Drops of Chocolate Syrup & Thin Slices of Strawberries

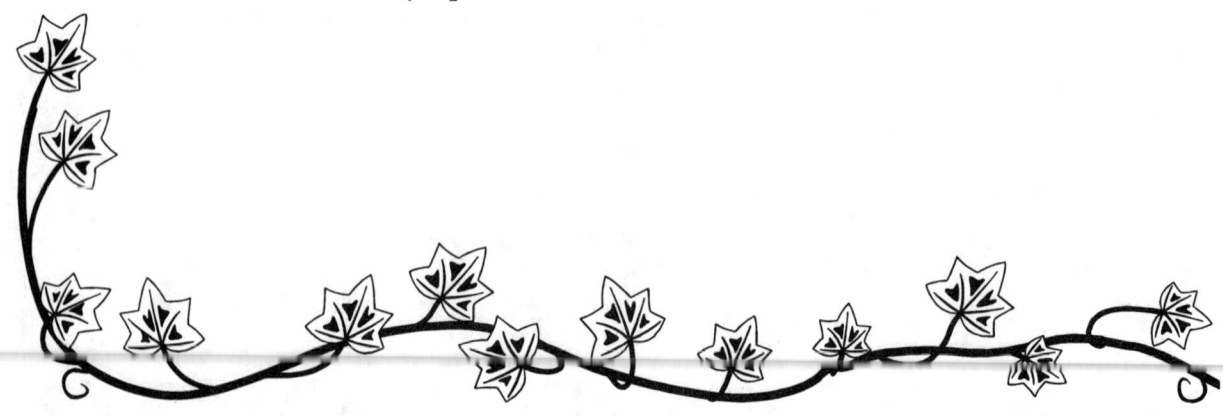

WEEK ONE - DAY # 5

Breakfast:
    Mother's Baked Egg Custard*
    3 Mini Muffins & Jam
    Chopped Fresh Fruits in season
    Non-fat Yogurt w/Honey
    Pear Juice
    Decaf Coffee

Mid-morning:
    Poached Prunes and Apricot Compote*

Lunch:
    Bay Shrimp Bisque* topped w/Herb Sprigs,
        serve warm w/soft crackers
    Mini Spinach Salad

Tea Time:
    Scones w/Honey & Jam
    Herb Tea

Dinner:
    The Hidden Garden Pasta w/Pesto*
    Chopped Fresh Tomato-Basil Salad

Evening Snack:
    Lemon Sorbet served in a frosted bowl
        w/mint leaf and cookie

WEEK ONE - DAY # 6

Breakfast:
    Poached Eggs
    Fan of Fresh Fruits: Kiwi, Berries, Pineapple
    Poppy Seed Almond Muffin & Jam
    Watermelon Juice
    Decaf Coffee

Mid-morning:
    ½ Cantaloupe
    Non-fat Yogurt w/Honey
    Warm Milk

Lunch:
    The Hidden Garden Chopped Salad*
        w/Paper-thin Slices of Turkey served
        w/Cucumber Dill Dressing
    Wheat Roll

Tea Time:
    Zangy Lemon Poppy Seed Cake*
    Herb Tea

Dinner:
    Baked Norwegian Salmon* served
        w/Wild Wild Rice*
        and Baked Japanese Eggplant,* garnished
        w/Sprigs of Parsley and Lemon Wedges

Evening Snack:
    Fresh Blueberries w/Creme Fraiche*

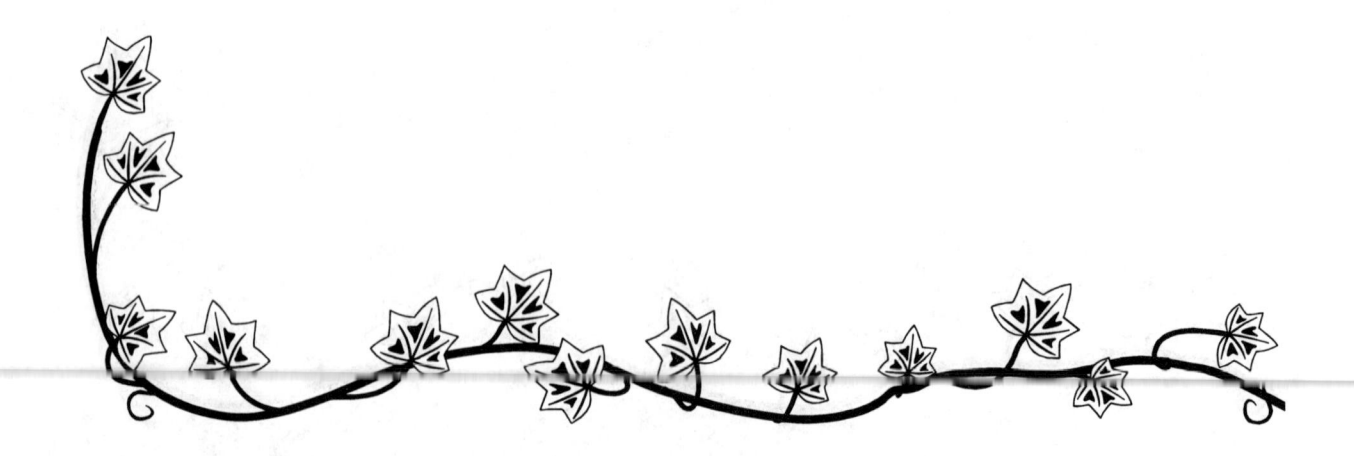

The Hollywood Facelift Diet

WEEK ONE - DAY # 7

Breakfast:	Cream of Wheat w/sprinkles of Brown Sugar
	Slices of Strawberries, Bananas and Grapes
	Scones w/Honey & Jam
	Non-fat Yogurt w/Honey
	Fresh Apple Juice
	Decaf Coffee
Mid-morning:	Diane's Fruit Smoothie*
Lunch:	Garden Fresh Chunky Vegetable Soup*
	Corn Bread
	Poached Pear* w/cinnamon stick
Tea Time:	Banana Fruit Tea Bread*
	Herbal Tea
Dinner:	Grandma Rocco's Pasta Primavera* elegantly garnished w/Italian Parsley & served w/Parmesan Cheese
Evening Snack:	Heavenly Chocolate Mousse w/Creme Fraiche* served with Raspberry Puree and a
	Mint Leaf

The Hollywood Facelift

WEEK TWO - DAY # 8

Breakfast:	Corn Muffin w/drops of Honey
	Large Fan of Fruits in season
	Fresh Cran/Apple Juice
	Non-fat Yogurt w/Honey
	Decaf Coffee
Mid-morning:	Poached Prunes and
	Apricot Compote*
Lunch:	Broccoli Soup* garnished
	w/Sprig of Parsley & Crackers
	Chopped Tomatoes
	Baked Apple
Tea Time:	Nola's Incredible 4th of July Apple Pie*
	Herbal Tea or Decaf Coffee
Dinner:	Paper Thin-sliced Chicken Picatta*
	with Fresh Garden Herbs served
	with fresh Baked Scallopini
	Squash with Dill*
	Dinner Roll
Evening Snack:	Nola's Incredible Blueberry Pie*
	Herb or Decaf Tea

Nola's Note: Can start to introduce *finely chopped* nuts and seeds, and carefully try citrus fruits. Chicken must be very thinly sliced.

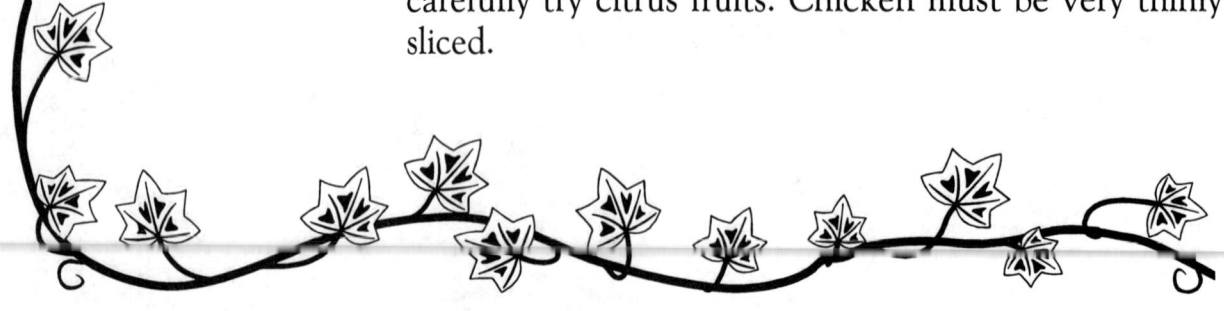

The Hollywood Facelift Diet

WEEK TWO - DAY # 9

Breakfast:	Grandmother's Oat Bran Mini-Muffin*
	Mango-Pineapple Juice
	Slices of Kiwi Fruit
	Non-fat Yogurt w/Honey
	Decaf Coffee
Mid-morning:	Fan of Freshly-Sliced Bananas and Strawberries w/Sprig of Mint
Lunch:	Fresh Tomato Mushroom Bisque*
	Australian Toast Muffin, lightly toasted
	Romaine Lettuce w/Pesto Sauce*
Tea Time:	Scones w/Honey & Jam
	Herbal Tea
Dinner:	Nola's Scampi and Herbs* sauteed in Olive Oil & Garlic and The Hidden Garden's Pasta w/Pesto* sprinkled w/Parmesan Cheese
Evening Snack:	Fresh Strawberries in a Parfait Topped w/Custard Sauce & Sprig of Mint
Nola's Note:	Australian Toast Muffins may be purchased at your local supermarket and they're softer than English Muffins.

WEEK TWO - DAY # 10

Breakfast:
    Pumpernickel Raisin Bread
        w/Whipped Light Cream Cheese
    Poached Pears*
    Non-fat Yogurt w/Drops of Honey
    Fresh Mango Juice
    Decaf Coffee/Tea

Mid-morning:
    ½ Cantaloupe w/Blueberries in center

Lunch:
    Fresh Fruit Platter elegantly garnished
        w/Italian Parsley and Low-fat Cottage Cheese

Tea Time:
    Sliced Zangy Lemon Poppy Seed Cake*
    Herb Tea

Dinner:
    Baked Chilean Sea Bass* served
        w/Fresh Tomato-Basil Salad,*
    Steamed Fresh Spinach w/drops of Olive Oil
    Baby White Potatoes Sauté w/Garlic &
        Chopped Parsley

Evening Snack:
    Teal's Chocolate-Chocolate-Chocolate Chip Cake*
        served warm topped with Vanilla Frozen Yogurt
    Herb or Decaf Tea

The Hollywood Facelift Diet

WEEK TWO - DAY # 11

Breakfast:	Warm Old-Fashioned Quaker Oats or Carrot Muffin Fan of Banana, Kiwi and Strawberries Non-fat Yogurt w/drops of honey or jam Pear Juice Decaf Coffee
Mid-morning:	Fresh Berries w/Custard Sauce*
Lunch:	Mushroom & Spinach Quiche Fresh Steamed Baby Carrots w/Dill Roll
Tea Time:	Raspberry Sorbet topped w/Fresh Raspberries

Dinner:	Chopped Turkey Sausage-Sweet Italian Style
	Special Italian Rigatoni Noodles*
	   w/Chopped Tomatoes & Herb Sauce
	Steamed Zucchini* brushed
	   w/Olive Oil and Fresh Basil

Evening Snack:	Nola's 4th of July Apple Pie* or Frozen Vanilla Yogurt

The Hollywood Facelift

WEEK TWO - DAY # 12

Breakfast:	Bowl of Chopped Fresh Fruit Salad
	Poached Eggs
	Lightly Toasted Wheat Bread & Fruit Preserve
	Non-fat Yogurt w/Drops of Honey
	Decaf Coffee
Mid-morning:	Slices of Fresh Watermelon
Lunch:	Cheese Omelette* Sprinkled w/Chives, elegantly garnish w/Sprigs of Parsley & Slices of Tomato
	Wheat Roll
Tea Time:	Slice of Carrot Cake, warmed
	Herb Tea or Café
Dinner:	Baked Cornish Game Hen* elegantly garnished w/Slices of Orange, Cucumber, Tomatoes & Parsley
	Wild Wild Rice*
Evening Snack:	Extra Dark Chocolate Brownies* w/Vanilla Non-Fat Ice Cream

Note: May return to "real" coffee and caffeine drinks at this time.

The Hollywood Facelift Diet

WEEK TWO - DAY # 13

Breakfast:	Scones w/Honey & Jam
	½ Cantaloupe w/Blueberries in center
	Non-fat Yogurt w/Honey drops
	Pear Juice
	Coffee
Mid-morning:	Stewed Prunes served in a Chilled Bowl
Lunch:	Garden Fresh Chunky Vegetable Soup
	Fresh Romaine Lettuce
	w/The Hidden Garden Pesto*
	Corn Bread
Tea Time:	Frozen Blueberry Yogurt w/Mint Leaf
Dinner:	Baked Norwegian Salmon* garnished with lemon
	Slices of Baked Japanese Eggplant*
	Baked Potato
Evening Snack:	Yummy Tapioca Pudding* w/Whole Strawberries

WEEK TWO - DAY # 14

Breakfast:
    Warm Mother's Baked Egg Custard*
    Large Fan of Fruits: Peaches, Kiwi, Bananas
    3 Mini Muffins/Honey & Jam
    Watermelon Juice
    Coffee

Mid-morning:
    Freshly Pureed Papaya w/Lemon

Lunch:
    The Hidden Garden Chopped Salad*
    Scoop of Chopped Chicken
       w/Cucumber Dill Dressing
    Wheat Roll

Tea Time:
    Vanilla Banana Milkshake

Dinner:
    The Hidden Garden Homemade
    Manicotti* w/Freshly Chopped
    Tomato and Herb sauce
    Baked Scallopini Squash* brushed
       w/Olive Oil and Dill Weed

Evening Snack:
    Poached Pear* on a chilled dessert plate
       w/Custard Sauce*
    Herbal Tea w/Honey

The Hollywood Facelift Diet

WEEK THREE - DAY # 15

Breakfast:	Poppy Seed Muffin/Honey & Jam
	Warm Chunky Style Applesauce
	w/Creme Fraiche*
	Fresh Pineapple Juice
	Coffee
Mid-morning:	Chilled ½ Fresh Papaya w/Lemon Slice
Lunch:	Open-faced Tuna Sandwich w/Choice of
	Thinly-Sliced Rye Bread or Croissant
	½ Cup Cantaloupe-Pineapple Soup
Tea Time:	Slice of Banana Fruit Tea Bread*
	Coffee or Tea
Dinner:	
	Sautéd Bay Scallops Royale*
	Steamed Asparagus served cold drizzled
	w/Cucumber Dill Dressing
Evening Snack:	Nola's Incredible Blueberry Pie*
	Cup of Tea or Coffee

The Hollywood Facelift

WEEK THREE - DAY # 16

Breakfast:	Croissants and Fruit Preserve
	Slices of Kiwi, Bananas & Grapes w/Yogurt
	Apple Juice
	Coffee
Mid-morning:	Strawberry-Banana Milkshake*
Lunch:	Fresh Tomato Mushroom Bisque*
	Fresh Spinach Salad w/choice of dressing
	Wheat Roll
Tea Time:	Lemon Poppy Seed Cake*
	Warm or Iced Herb Tea
Dinner:	Grandma Rocco's Pasta Primavera* elegantly garnished w/Italian Parsley & served w/Parmesan Cheese
Evening Snack:	Lemon Sorbet w/Mint Sprig

The Hollywood Facelift Diet

WEEK THREE - DAY # 17

Breakfast:	Poached Eggs
	Slightly Toasted Honey-Wheat Bread
	Jam
	Choice of Juice
	Fresh Strawberries
Mid-morning:	Stewed Prunes w/Lemon
Lunch:	Homemade Broccoli Soup*
	Bowl of Chopped Fresh Fruit Salad
	Wheat Roll
Tea Time:	Nola's Incredible Blueberry Pie*
	Herb Tea
Dinner:	Broiled Chilean Sea Bass*
	served w/Fresh Tomato-Basil Salad*
	"Real" Italian Country Style Polenta*
	Steamed Fresh Spinach w/drops of Olive Oil
Evening Snack:	Lowfat Chocolate Ice Cream on an Old-Fashioned Sugar Cone

WEEK THREE - DAY # 18

Breakfast:
    Mother's Oat Bran Cereal
    Poached Prunes and Apricot Compote*
    Fresh Mango-Pineapple Juice
    Coffee

Mid-morning:
    Fresh Poached Pear* garnished w/Cinnamon Stick

Lunch:
    Chilled Cantaloupe-Pineapple Soup
        w/Sprig of Mint
    Thin Slices of Avocado on a bed of lettuce
        with tomato slices and goat cheese
    Wheat Crackers

Tea Time:
    Scones w/Honey & Jam
    Tea

Dinner:
    Chicken Picatta* with Fresh Garden Herbs
    Slices of Tomato
    Steamed Zucchini* with Fresh Basil

Evening Snack:
    Teal's Chocolate-Chocolate-Chocolate Chip Cake*

The Hollywood Facelift Diet

WEEK THREE - DAY # 19

Breakfast:	Scones w/Honey & Fruit Preserve Fresh Berries w/Mint and Yogurt Fresh Apricot Juice Coffee
Mid-morning:	Baked Apple w/Custard Sauce*

Lunch:	Mushroom & Spinach Quiche
	    w/Steamed Whole Baby Carrots brushed
	    w/Oil and Dill
	Wheat Roll

Tea Time:	Slice of Cranberry Tea Bread Herb Tea

Dinner:	Nola's Scampi and Herbs*
	    sauted in Olive Oil and Garlic
	The Hidden Garden Pasta w/Pesto*
	    sprinkled with Parmesan Cheese
	Fresh Tomato-Basil Salad*

Evening Snack:	Strawberry Sorbet and a Cookie

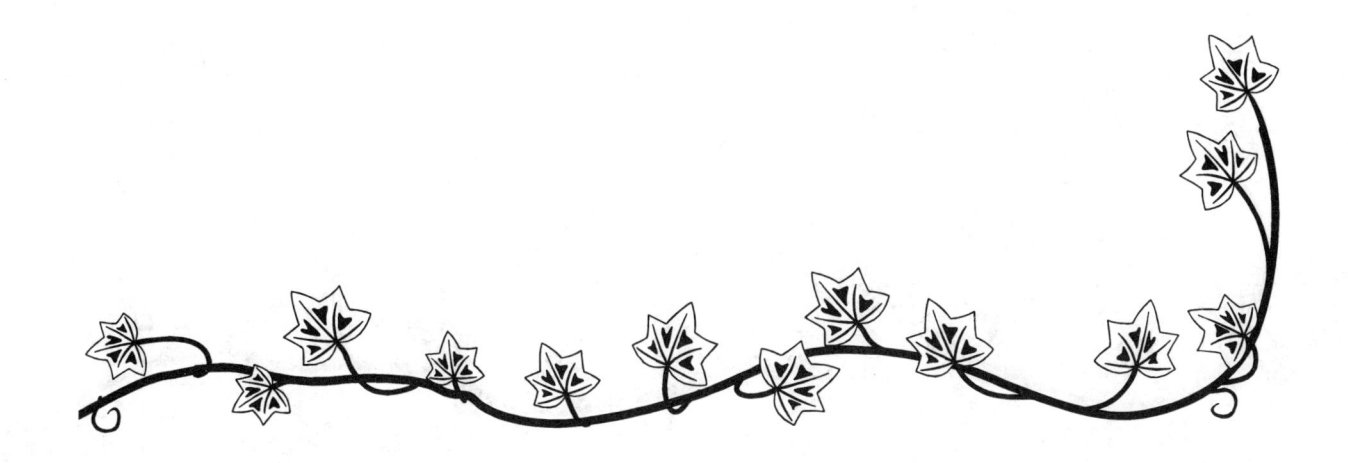

WEEK THREE - DAY # 20

Breakfast:
    Freshly Chopped Fruits in Season
        topped w/Non-fat Cottage Cheese
    Fresh Pear Juice
    Coffee

Mid-morning:
    Diane's Fruit Smoothie*

Lunch:
    The Hidden Garden Chopped Salad*
        w/Chopped Turkey
    Choice of dressing
    ½ cup Shrimp Bisque*
    Wheat Roll

Tea Time:
    Slice of Carrot Cake
    Coffee or Tea

Dinner:
    Baked Norwegian Salmon* served
        w/Steamed Broccoli or
        Baked Japanese Eggplant*
    Baked Potato or Wild Wild Rice*

Evening Snack:
    Heavenly Chocolate Mousse*
        with Creme Fraiche*
        and Slices or Whole Strawberries

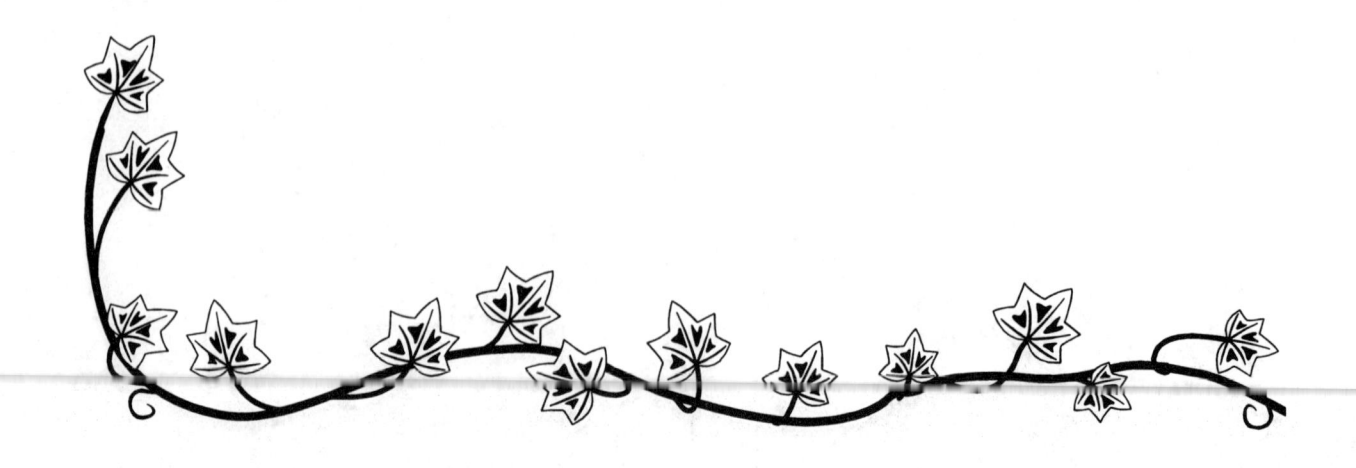

The Hollywood Facelift Diet

WEEK THREE - DAY # 21

Breakfast:	Grandmother's Oat Bran Mini Muffin*
	Honey & Jam
	Poached Pear*
	Fresh Cran/Apple Juice
	Coffee

Mid-morning:	Non-fat Plain Yogurt w/Chopped Stewed Prunes

Lunch:	Spinach Omelette
	½ cup of Cantaloupe-Pineapple Soup*
	Wheat Roll

Tea Time:	Wafer Cookies
	Warm or Iced Tea

Dinner:	Cornish Game Hen* elegantly garnished
	    w/Slices of Orange, Cucumber,
	    Tomatoes & Parsley
	Bed of Wild Wild Rice* or
	"Real" Italian Country Style Polenta*

Evening Snack:	Nola's 4th of July Apple Pie* served warm
	    w/Scoop of Non-Fat Vanilla Ice Cream

WEEK FOUR - DAY # 22

Breakfast:
    Scrambled Egg Whites w/White Pepper
    Croissant and Jam
    Chilled Mandarin Orange Slices
    Fresh Apricot Juice
    Coffee

Mid-morning:
    Fan of Freshly-Sliced Bananas, Kiwi and Melon

Lunch:
    Open-faced Tuna Sandwich on a bed of Lettuce
        w/Slices of Tomatoes
    Choice of Rye or Wheat Bread

Tea Time:
    Dr. Fisher's Milkshake*

Dinner:
    Fresh Special Italian Rigatoni Noodles*
        w/Tomato-Basil Sauce sprinkled
        w/Parmesan Cheese and
        served w/Baked Scallopini Green Squash*
    Brushed w/Olive Oil and Dill

Evening Snack:
    Fresh Blueberries with Creme Fraiche*
        and a Mint Leaf

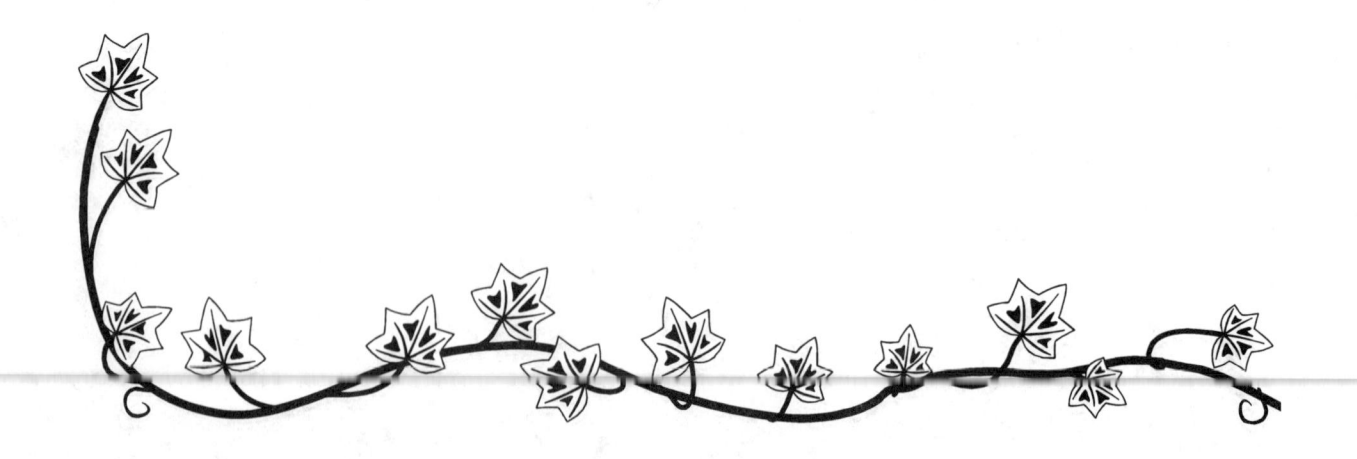

The Hollywood Facelift Diet

WEEK FOUR - DAY # 23

Breakfast:	Scones w/Honey and Jam
	Poached Prunes and Apricot Compote*
	Mango/Pineapple Juice
	Coffee
Mid-morning:	Poached Pear* served w/Cinnamon Stick
Lunch:	Goat Cheese Omelette*
	sprinkled w/Freshly Chopped Parsley &
	served w/Slices of Grapes & Kiwi
	Fresh Romaine Lettuce with
	The Hidden Garden Pesto Sauce*
	Wheat Roll
Tea Time:	Blueberry Milkshake
	Warm English Tea w/Honey
Dinner:	Chopped Turkey Sausage-Sweet Italian Style
	Pasta w/Olive Oil and Garlic
	Fresh Tomato Basil Salad*
Evening Snack:	Extra Dark Chocolate Brownies*
	sliced & served warm w/ Non-Fat Ice Cream

The Hollywood Facelift

WEEK FOUR - DAY # 24

Breakfast:	Cream of Wheat w/sprinkles of Brown Sugar
	Australian Toast Muffin, lightly toasted, with Jam
	Non-fat Yogurt w/Fresh Berries and Honey
	Papaya Puree
	Coffee
Mid-morning:	Slices of Fresh Watermelon
Lunch:	Quiche, baked & served w/Mini Wheat Croissant
	½ cup Carrot Soup
Tea Time:	Lemon Sorbet and Mint Cookies
Dinner:	Sauteed Bay Scallops Royale*
	in Olive Oil, Garlic & Lemon
	sprinkled w/Herbs and
	garnished w/Slices of Lemon & Parsley
	Fresh Chopped Spinach Salad
	½ Baked Potato
Evening Snack:	Teal's Chocolate-Chocolate-Chocolate Chip Cake served warm!
	Topped with cook's choice!

The Hollywood Facelift Diet

WEEK FOUR - DAY # 25

Breakfast:	Poached Eggs
Bowl of Freshly-Sliced Fruits
topped w/Cottage Cheese
Honey Wheat Toast w/Fruit Preserve
Fresh Pineapple Juice
Coffee
Mid-morning:	Chilled Bowl of Blueberries w/Custard Sauce
Lunch:	The Hidden Garden Chopped Salad*
w/Chicken White Meat and Slices of Avocado
Cup of The Hidden Garden Homemade
Bay Shrimp Bisque*
Wheat Roll or Slice of Rye
Tea Time:	Nola's 4th of July Apple Pie*
Herbal Tea
Dinner:	Homemade Manicotti* w/Slices of Steamed
Green Scallopini Squash*
Evening Snack:	Lemon Sorbet in chilled bowl
garnished w/Mint Leaf

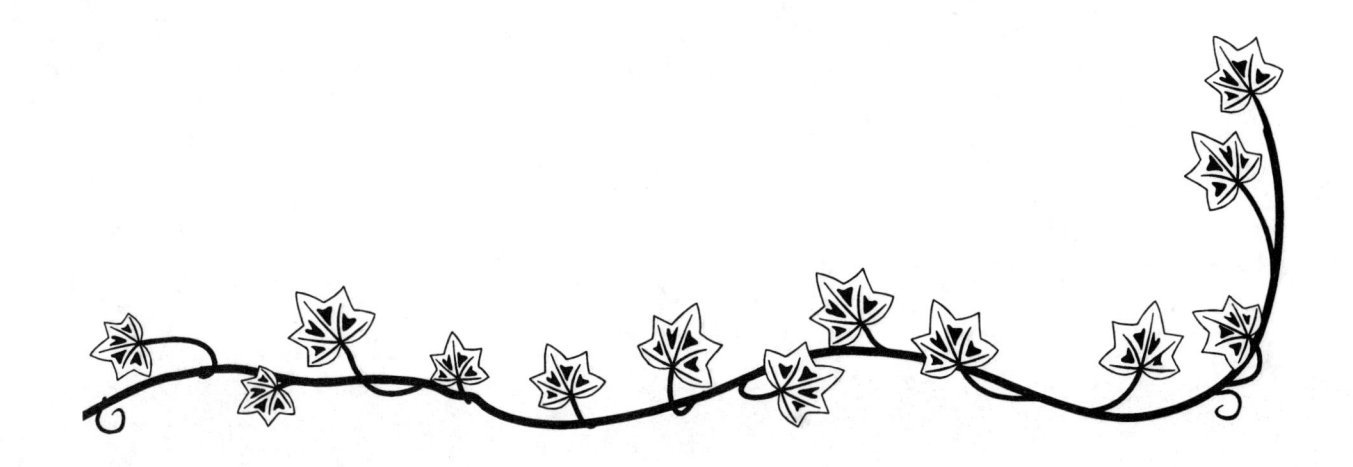

WEEK FOUR - DAY # 26

Breakfast:
        Poached Prunes and Apricot Compote*
        Mini Muffins w/Honey and Jam
        Fresh Mango-Pineapple Juice
        Coffee

Mid-morning:
        Baked Apple sprinkled w/Brown Sugar

Lunch:
        Mushroom Omelette* sprinkled w/Chopped Chives
            & elegantly garnished w/Italian Parsley
        Slices of Tomatoes & Mint Cucumber Salad
        Toast

Tea Time:
        Slice of Banana Fruit Tea Bread*
        Warm English Tea

Dinner:
        Broiled Chilean Sea Bass*
            w/ Fresh Tomato-Basil Salad*
        Baked Yam or
        "Real" Italian Country Style Polenta*

Evening Snack:
        Vanilla Ice Cream Drizzled w/Chocolate Syrup
            w/Mint Leaf and a Wafer Cookie

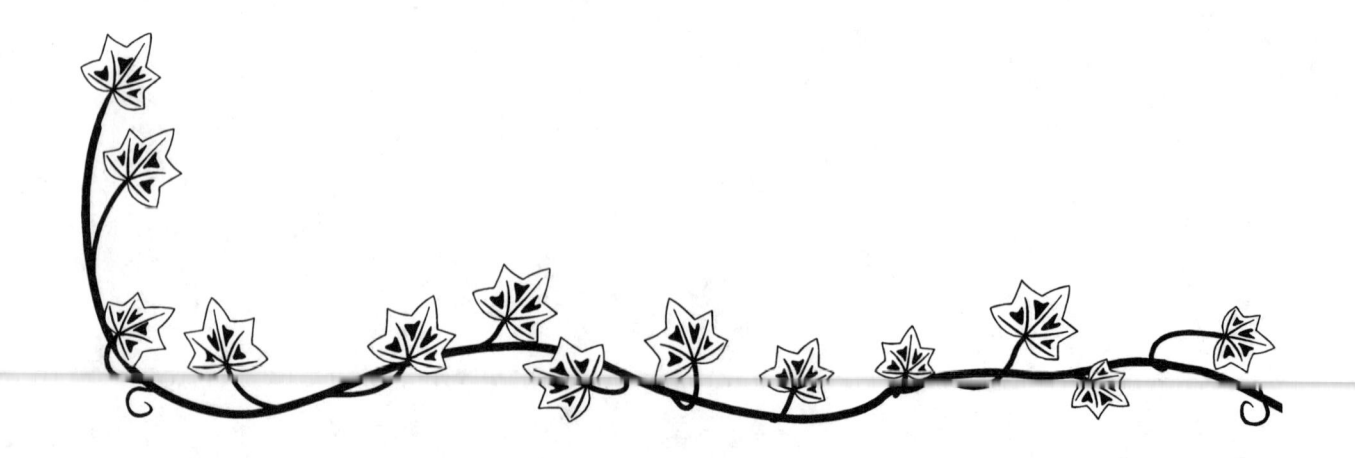

The Hollywood Facelift Diet

WEEK FOUR - DAY # 27

Breakfast:	Warm Mother's Baked Egg Custard* Poppy Seed Muffin w/Honey Mango-Pineapple Slices Coffee
Mid-morning:	Poached Prunes and Apricot Compote*
Lunch:	Hidden Garden Homemade Potato Soup* Fruit Platter Wheat Roll
Tea Time:	Nola's Incredible Homemade Blueberry Pie* Tea or Coffee

Dinner:	Thinly-Sliced Chicken Picatta*
	    with Fresh Garden Herbs served hot
	    w/Baked Japanese Eggplant*
	    and Tomato-Basil Salad*

Evening Snack:	Chilled Bowl of Fresh Strawberries w/Custard Sauce*

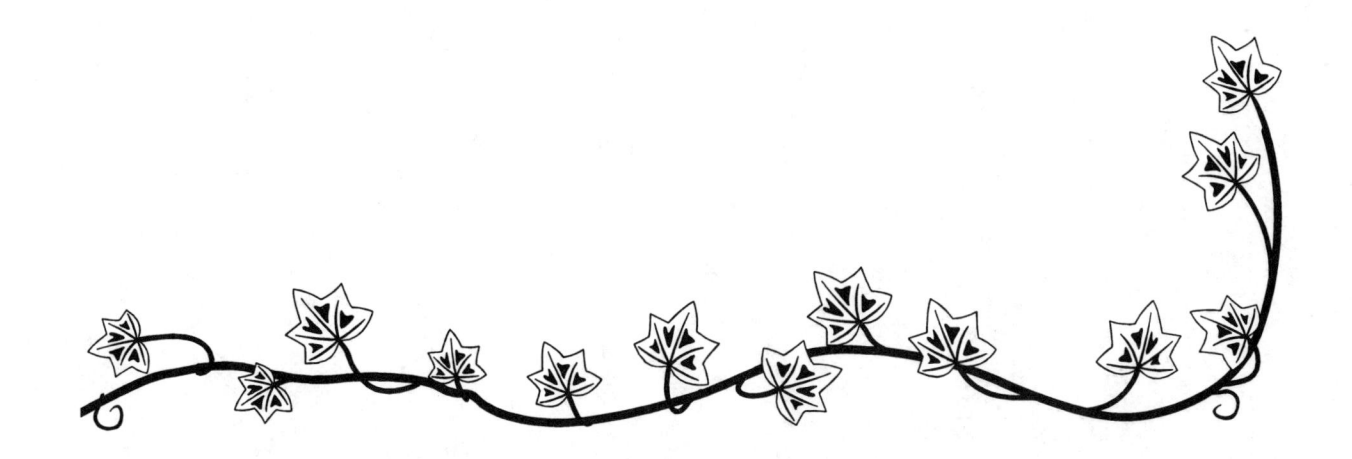

WEEK FOUR - DAY # 28

Breakfast:	Papaya Puree
	Blueberry Muffin & Fruit Preserve
	Nonfat Yogurt w/Drops of Honey
	Coffee
Mid-morning:	Fresh Pear Sliced Thin
	w/Slice of Goat Cheese
Lunch:	Mushroom Tomato Bisque*
	Mint Cucumber Salad*
	Slice of Wheat Grain Bread
Tea Time:	Herbal Tea
	Slice of Zangy Lemon Poppy Seed Cake*
Dinner:	Nola's Scampi and Herbs*
	Sauteed in Olive Oil and Garlic
	The Hidden Garden Pasta* w/Pesto*
	sprinkled w/Parmesan Cheese
Evening Snack:	Fresh Blueberries chilled w/Creme Fraiche*

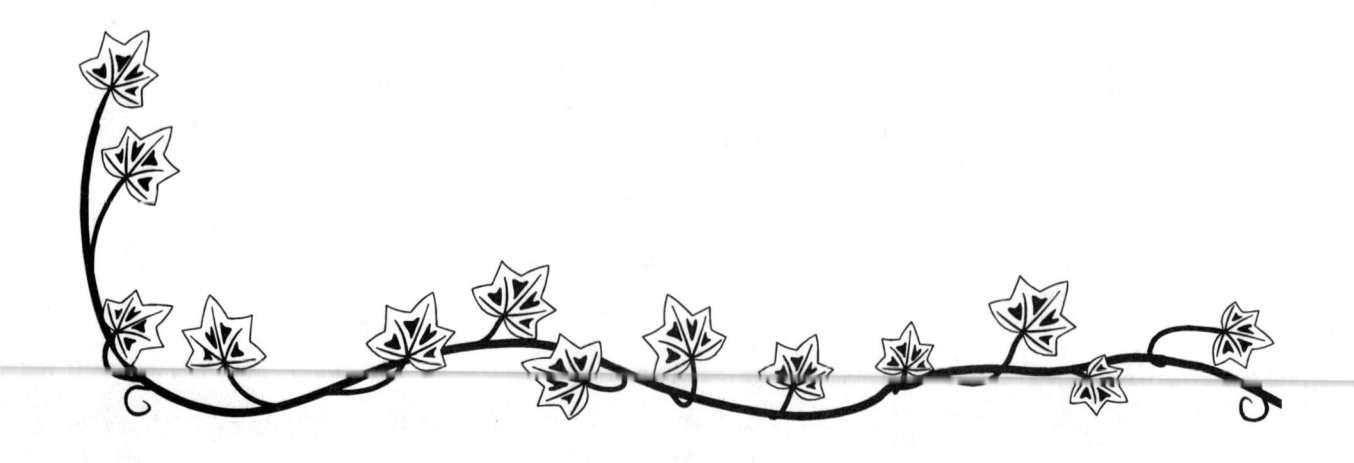

The Hollywood Facelift Diet

For Peel/Dermabrasion/Tummy Tuck

DAY # 1

Arrival: Diane's Fruit Smoothie*

Dinner: Hidden Garden Homemade Chicken Broth*
                     Fresh Fruit Juices

Evening Snack: Blueberry Milkshake*

Nola's Note: Strictly Liquid Diet!

For Peel/Dermabrasion/Tummy Tuck

DAY # 2

Breakfast: Strawberry-Banana Milkshake*
                      Decaf

Mid-morning: Fresh Mango Puree

Lunch: Vegetable Protein Powder Shake
                      Cran/Applesauce

Tea Time: Soft Fruit Flavored Jello

Dinner: Country Inn Potato Leek Soup*
                          served warm w/Sprig of Parsley
                      Fresh Fruit Juice

Evening Snack: Chocolate Milkshake*

The Hollywood Facelift Diet

For Peel/Dermabrasion/Tummy Tuck

DAY # 3

Breakfast:	Milk & Egg Protein Powder Shake
Mid-morning:	Cool & Pure Pear Juice
Lunch:	The Hidden Garden Homemade Carrot Soup* Cantaloupe puree
Tea Time:	Diane's Fruit Smoothie*
Dinner:	Large bowl of Bay Shrimp Bisque* Fresh Juice
Evening Snack:	Blueberry Milkshake*

For Peel/Dermabrasion/Tummy Tuck

DAY # 4

Breakfast:
    Cream of Wheat w/sprinkles of Brown Sugar
    Mother's Baked Egg Custard*
    Finely-Chopped Fruit Salad:
        Grapes, Strawberries, Melon
    Nonfat Plain Yogurt w/Drops of Honey
    Pineapple Juice
    Decaf Coffee

Mid-morning:
    Zesty Kiwi Slices

Lunch:
    Broccoli Soup*
    Soft Crackers
    Chilled Mango Puree

Tea Time:
    Dr. Fisher's Milkshake*

Dinner:
    Fresh Tomato-Mushroom Bisque*
    Wheat Crackers
    Mashed Potatoes

Evening Snack:
    Chilled Raspberry Sorbet and Cookie

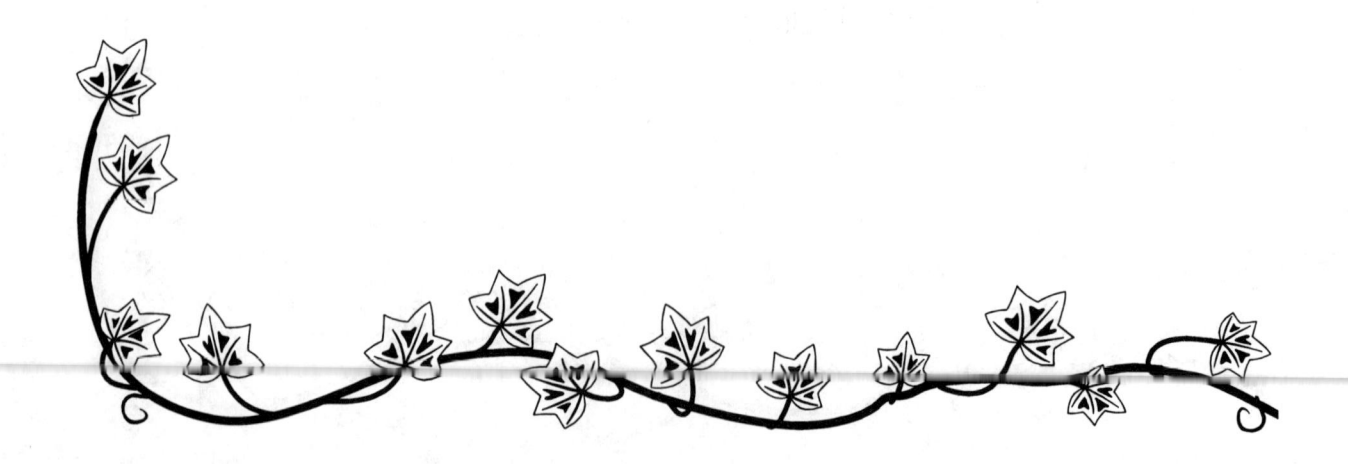

The Hollywood Facelift Diet

For Peel/Dermabrasion/Tummy Tuck

DAY # 5

Breakfast:	Scrambled Egg Whites w/ White Pepper Nonfat Plain Yogurt w/Honey Poached Pear Mango Juice Decaf Coffee
Mid-morning:	Wafer Cookies
Lunch:	Garden Fresh Chunky Vegetable Soup* Wheat Crackers Bowl of Chopped Fruits in season
Tea Time:	Slice of Banana Fruit Tea Bread* Iced Herbal Tea

Dinner:	The Hidden Garden Homemade Manicotti*
	   w/freshly-chopped tomato and herb sauce
	Baked Scallopini Squash brushed
	   w/Olive Oil and Dill Weed*

Evening Snack:	Yummy Tapioca Pudding* served warm or cold

Continue with Day #6 of
The Hidden Garden Facelift Diet

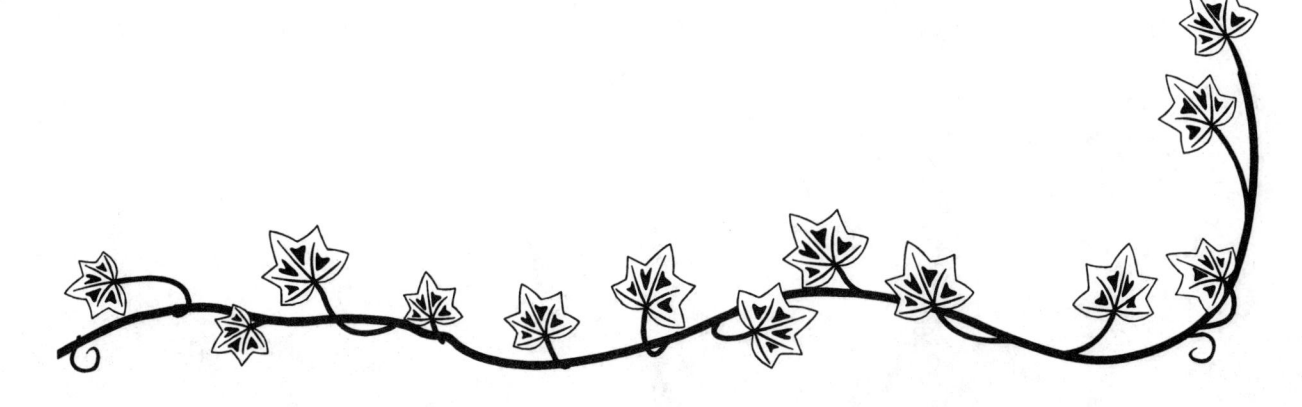

The Hollywood Facelift

For Liposuction

DAY # 1

Arrival: Slices of Banana
       Gatorade Drinks

Dinner: The Hidden Garden Homemade Chicken Soup*
        w/Chopped Carrots, Shredded Chicken
       and Angel's Hair Noodles
       Baked Potato
       Wheat Roll

Evening Snack: Yummy Tapioca Pudding* served warm or cold,
        or Frozen Blueberry Yogurt

Midnight: Strawberry-Banana Milkshake*

Nola's Note: Having Liposuction is just like running a 10K. Food and drinks high in potassium are important now.

The Hollywood Facelift Diet

For Liposuction

DAY #2

Breakfast:	Croissants/Fruit Preserve
	Mother's Baked Egg Custard*
	Nonfat Plain Yogurt w/Honey
	Fresh Mango-Pineapple-Banana Juice
	Decaf Coffee
Mid-morning:	Poached Pear* w/Cinnamon Sticks
	Gatorade Drinks
Lunch:	Bay Shrimp Bisque*
	Crackers or Roll
	Fresh Romaine Lettuce
	with The Hidden Garden Pesto*
Tea Time:	Poached Prunes and Apricot Compote*
Dinner:	The Hidden Garden Homemade Manicotti*
	w/freshly chopped Tomatoes & Herb Sauce
	served w/Baked Scallopini Squash*
Evening Snack:	Blueberry Milkshake*
	served in a Parfait and Cookie

The Hollywood Facelift

For Liposuction

DAY # 3

Breakfast:	Scrambled or Poached Eggs
	Honey Wheat Toast/Fruit Preserve
	Large Fan of Kiwi, Banana & Strawberries
	Pear Juice
	Decaf
Mid-morning:	Zesty Mango Puree in a chilled bowl
Lunch:	The Hidden Garden Chopped Salad*
	w/scoop of Tuna served
	w/Cucumber Dill Dressing
	Wheat Roll
Tea Time:	Slice of Nola's Incredible Blueberry Pie*
	Herbal Tea
Dinner:	Thinly-sliced Chicken Picatta*
	with Fresh Garden Herbs
	elegantly garnished w/slices of Lemon,
	Tomatoes & Baked Japanese Eggplant*
	Dinner Roll
Evening Snack:	Raspberry Sorbet

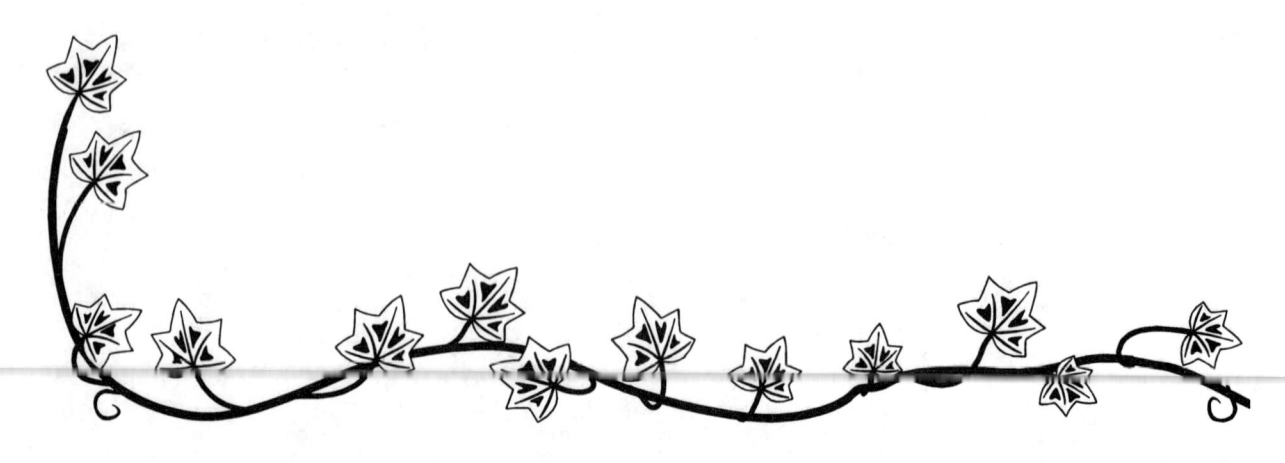

The Hollywood Facelift Diet

For Liposuction

DAY # 4

Breakfast:	Warm Old-Fashioned Quaker Oats Croissant/Honey and Jam Bowl of Fruits: Melon, Grapes, Pineapple Nonfat Plain Yogurt w/Honey Mango Juice Decaf Coffee
Mid-morning:	Baked Apple Cup of Decaf or Herbal Tea
Lunch:	The Hidden Garden Chopped Salad* w/slices of Turkey Wheat Roll ½ cup of Homemade Cantaloupe-Pineapple Soup*
Tea Time:	Slice of Lemon Poppy Seed Cake* Cup of Herbal Tea
Dinner:	Broiled Chilean Sea Bass* served w/chopped Fresh Tomato-Basil Salad* Steamed Zucchini* Baked Yam
Evening Snack:	Frozen Vanilla Yogurt w/ drops of Chocolate Syrup and Slices of Strawberries

The Hollywood Facelift

For Liposuction

DAY # 5

Breakfast:	Grandmother's Oat Bran Muffin/Honey
Fresh Strawberries w/Custard Sauce
Nonfat Plain Yogurt
Pear Juice
Decaf

Mid-morning:	Slices of Watermelon or Fruit in season

Lunch:	Spinach Omelette* sprinkled w/chopped Parsley
    and slices of Tomatoes
Wheat Toast

Tea Time:	Slice of Nola's 4th of July Apple Pie*
Herb Tea

Dinner:	Baked Norwegian Salmon*
    served with sautéed Wild Wild rice*
    or Baked Potato garnished with parsley
Baked Japanese Eggplant*

Evening Snack:	Chocolate Mousse* w/Creme Fraiche*
    served with fresh Raspberries

Continue with Day #6 of
The Hidden Garden Facelift Diet

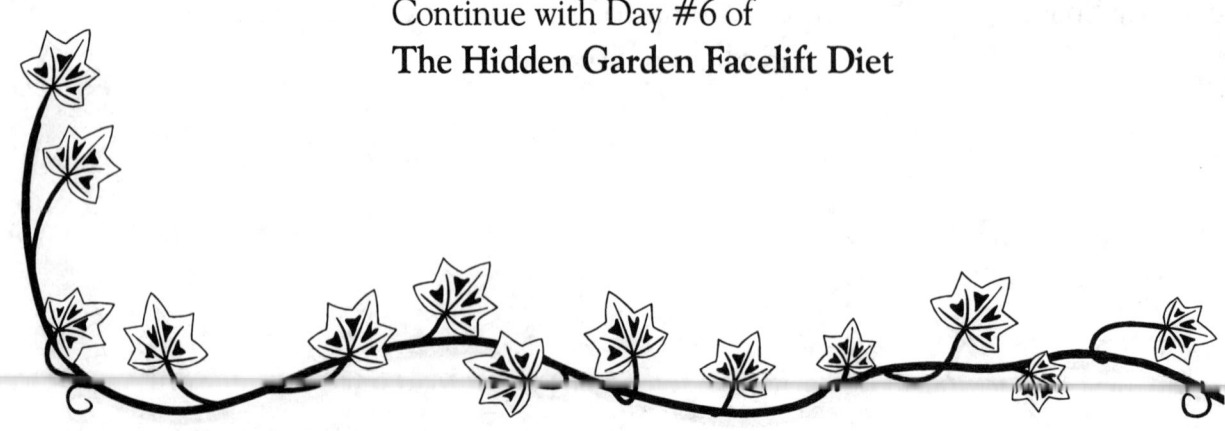

The Hollywood Facelift Diet

For Nasal Surgery Patients - Soft Diet

DAY # 1

Arrival:	Diane's Fruit Smoothie*
	Apple/Cranberry Sauce
Dinner:	Hidden Garden Homemade Chicken Soup *
	Mashed Potatoes
	Fresh Juice
Evening Snack:	Zesty Mango Purée
Midnight:	Raspberry Sorbet or Blueberry Milkshake
	(use soya milk)

Nola's Note: Soft Diet!
No Milk Products!
No Hot or Cold Foods!

Many doctors do not like their patients "sucking" on a straw. ASK!

The Hollywood Facelift

For Nasal Surgery Patients

DAY # 2

Breakfast:	Warm Cream of Wheat w/sprinkles of Brown Sugar Pear Juice
Mid-morning:	Zesty Mango Puree
Lunch:	The Hidden Garden Homemade Carrot Soup* served warm w/Sprig of Parsley Wheat Crackers Apple Sauce
Tea Time:	Protein Powder Shake (use soya milk)
Dinner:	Country Inn Potato-Leek Soup* Soft Crackers
Evening Snack:	Diane's Fruit Smoothie*

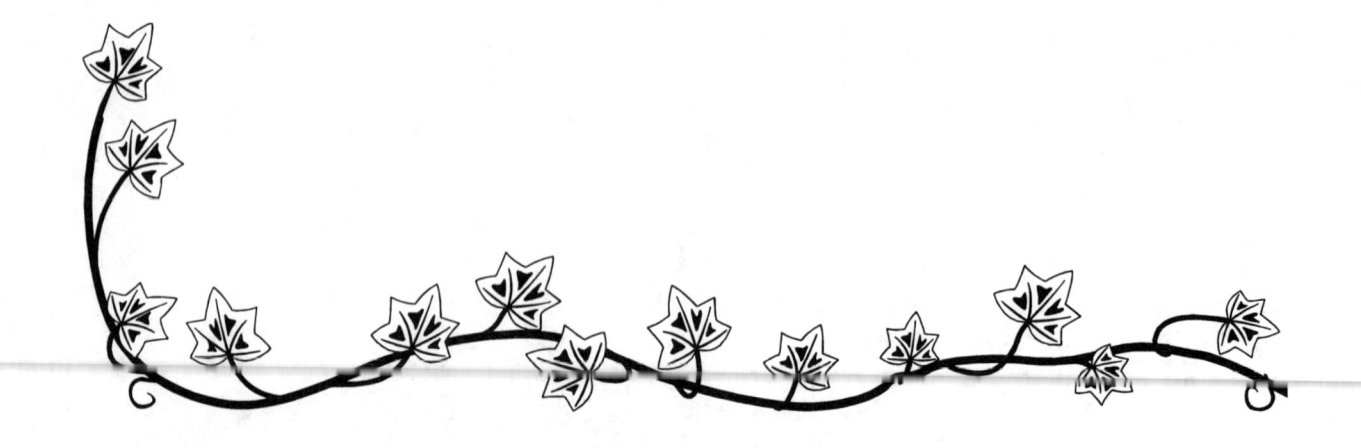

The Hollywood Facelift Diet

For Nasal Surgery Patients

DAY # 3

Breakfast:	Poached Egg Applesauce Fan of Bananas, Kiwi and Strawberries Mango/Pineapple Juice
Mid-morning:	Lemon Sorbet
Lunch:	Fresh Tomato Mushroom Bisque* served warm sprinkled with Chopped Scallions
Tea Time:	Poached Pear*
Dinner:	Cheese or Spinach Omelette* Banana Squash pureed
Evening Snacks:	Strawberry Sorbet w/crushed fresh strawberries

The Hollywood Facelift

For Nasal Surgery Patients

DAY # 4

Breakfast:	Warm Old-Fashioned Quaker Oats
	Finely-chopped Grapes, Strawberries and Melon
	Fresh Pear Juice
	Decaf Coffee or Tea
Mid-morning:	Zesty Kiwi Slices
	Herb Tea
Lunch:	Homemade Potato Leek Soup* and Soft Crackers
	Mango Puree
Tea Time:	Strawberry-Banana Shake* (use soya milk)
Dinner:	Broiled Chilean Sea Bass*
	served with Baked Yam and
	finely-chopped Fresh Basil-Tomato-Basil Salad*
Evening Snacks:	Raspberry Sorbet and a Soft Cookie

The Hollywood Facelift Diet

For Nasal Surgery Patients

DAY # 5

Breakfast:	3 Mini Soft Muffins/Honey & Jam
	Poached Pear*
	Apricot Juice
	Decaf Coffee
Mid-morning:	Warm Decaf Tea
	Wafer Cookies
Lunch:	Chilled Cantaloupe-Pineapple Soup*
	Scoop of Tuna Salad (no lettuce)
	Wheat Rolls
Tea Time:	A Slice of Banana Fruit Tea Bread*
	Warm Herbal Tea
Dinner:	The Hidden Garden Homemade Manicotti*
	w/freshly chopped Tomato and Herb Sauce
	Steamed Zucchini* with Basil
	garnished with sprig of parsley
Evening Snacks:	Lemon Sorbet w/mint leaf

Continue with Day #6 of
The Hidden Garden Facelift Diet

The Hidden Garden Cookbook

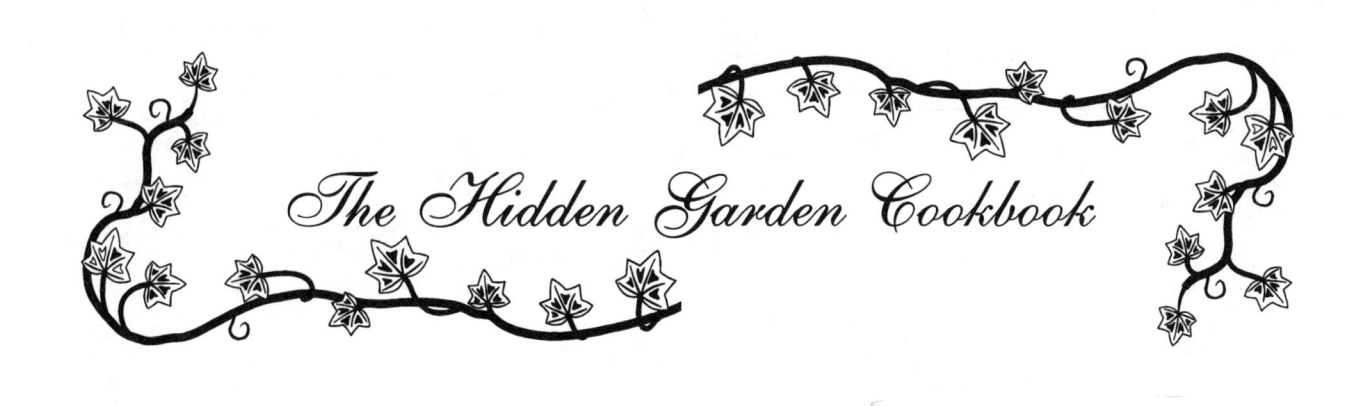

Part 3

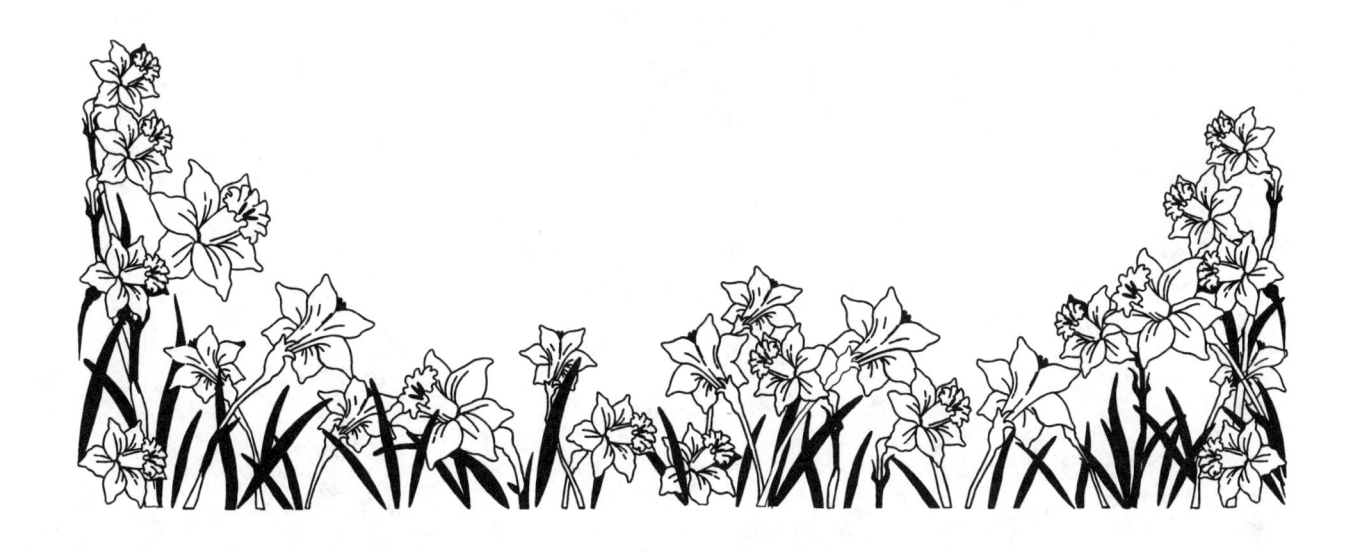

The Hidden Garden Cookbook

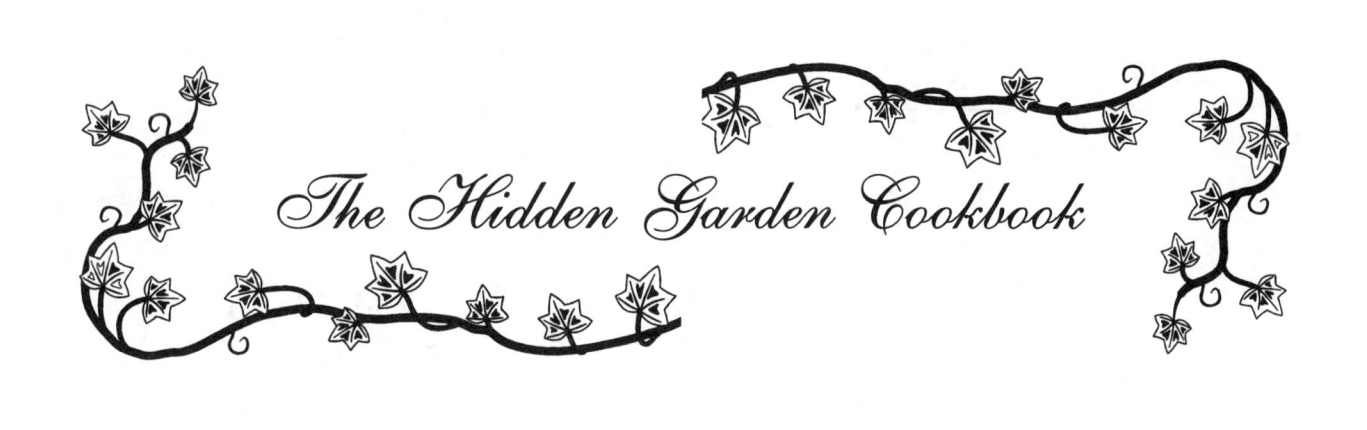

Salad

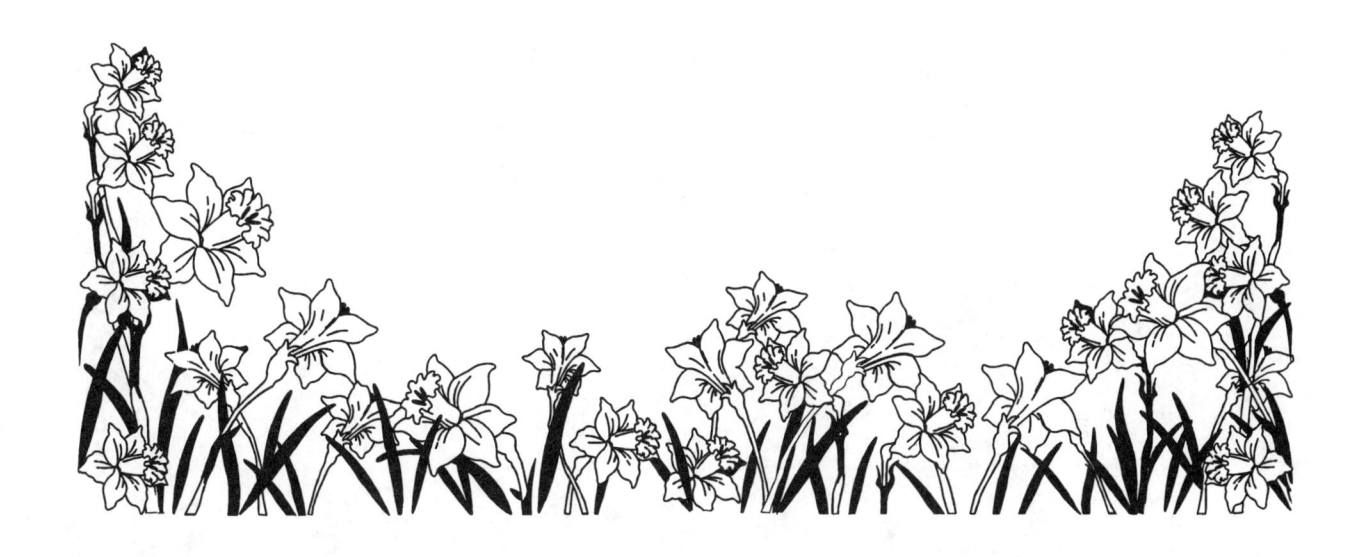

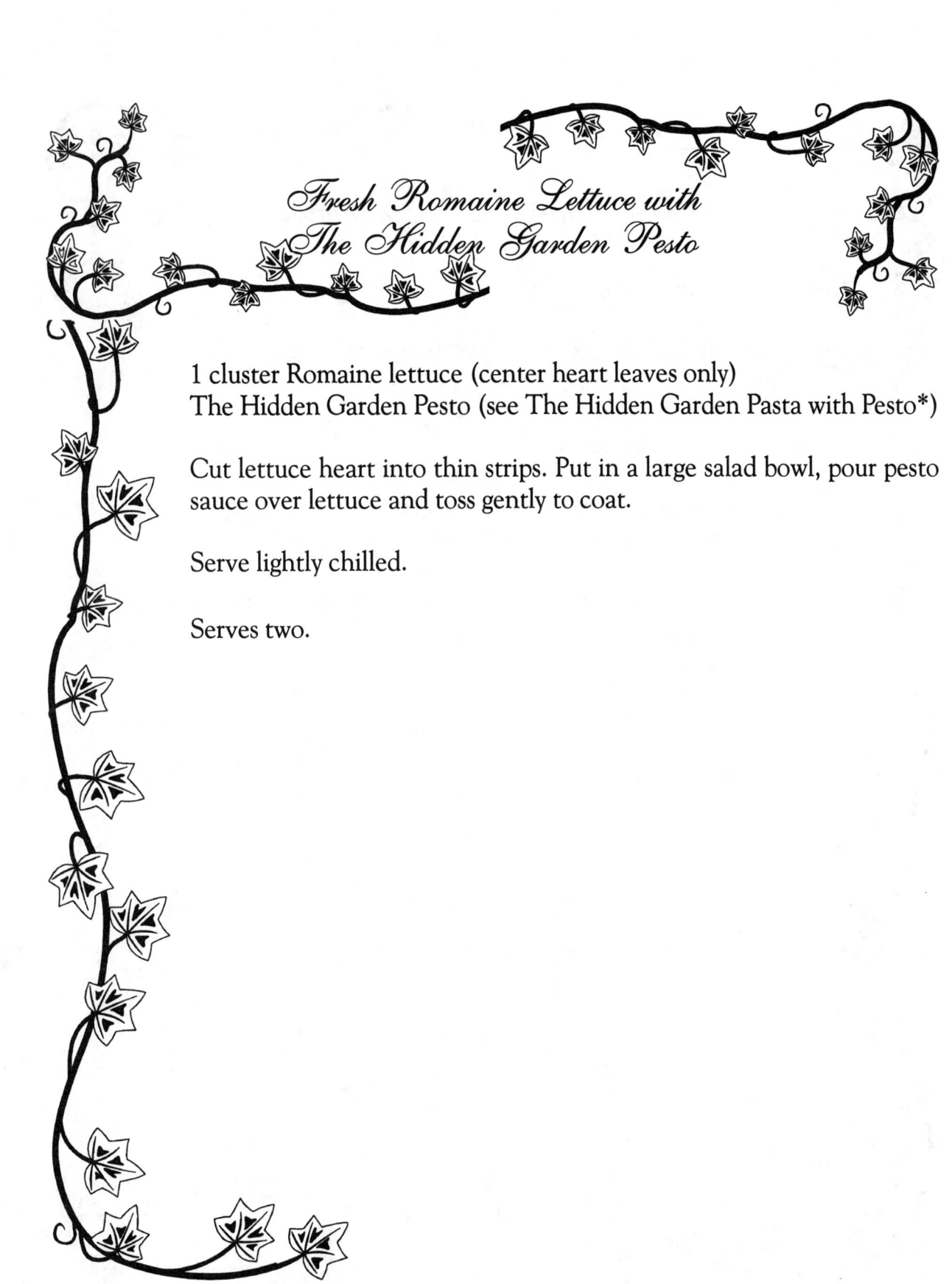

Fresh Romaine Lettuce with The Hidden Garden Pesto

1 cluster Romaine lettuce (center heart leaves only)
The Hidden Garden Pesto (see The Hidden Garden Pasta with Pesto*)

Cut lettuce heart into thin strips. Put in a large salad bowl, pour pesto sauce over lettuce and toss gently to coat.

Serve lightly chilled.

Serves two.

Fresh Basil - Tomato Salad

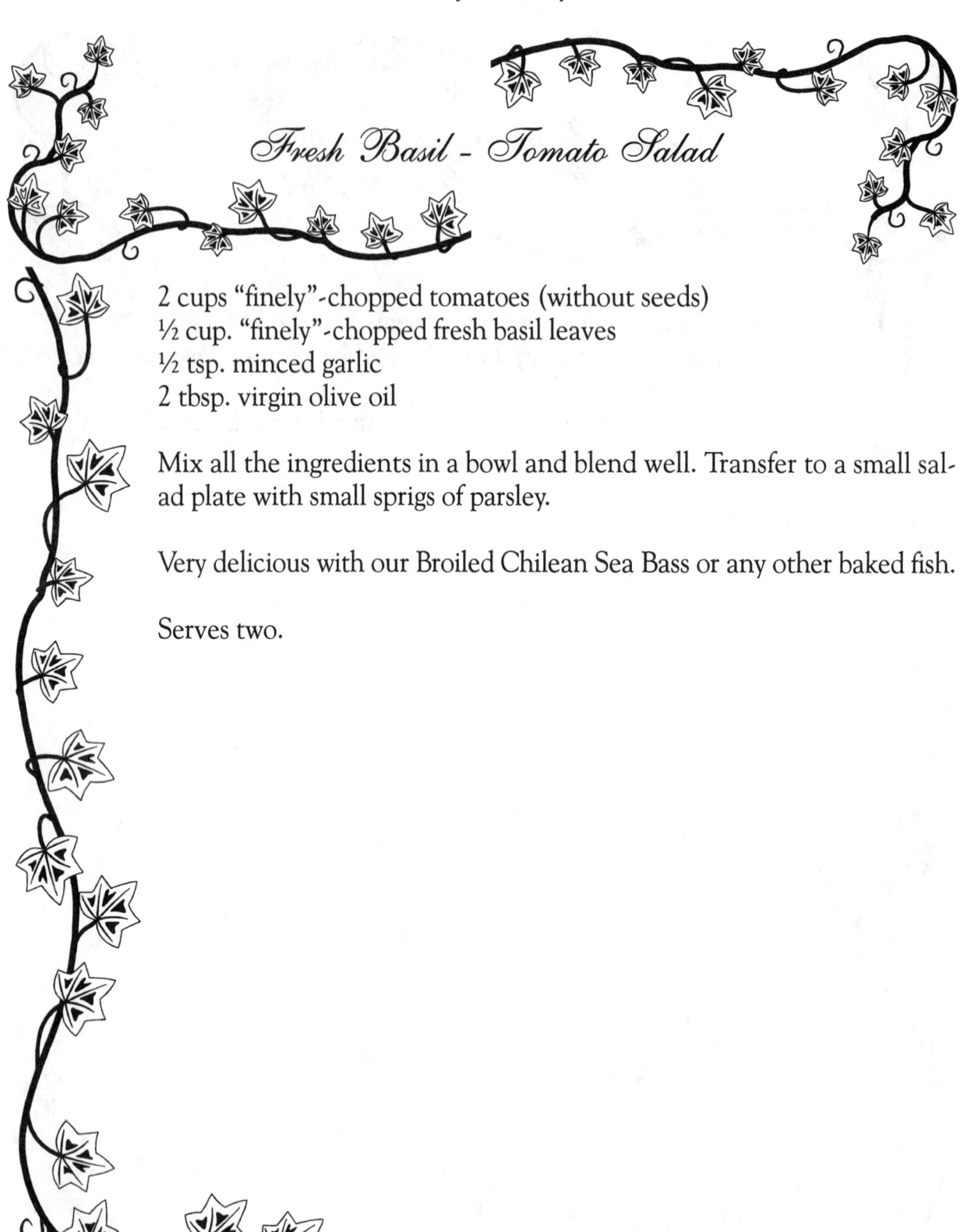

2 cups "finely"-chopped tomatoes (without seeds)
½ cup. "finely"-chopped fresh basil leaves
½ tsp. minced garlic
2 tbsp. virgin olive oil

Mix all the ingredients in a bowl and blend well. Transfer to a small salad plate with small sprigs of parsley.

Very delicious with our Broiled Chilean Sea Bass or any other baked fish.

Serves two.

The Hidden Garden Chopped Salad
(with Tuna, Chicken or Turkey)

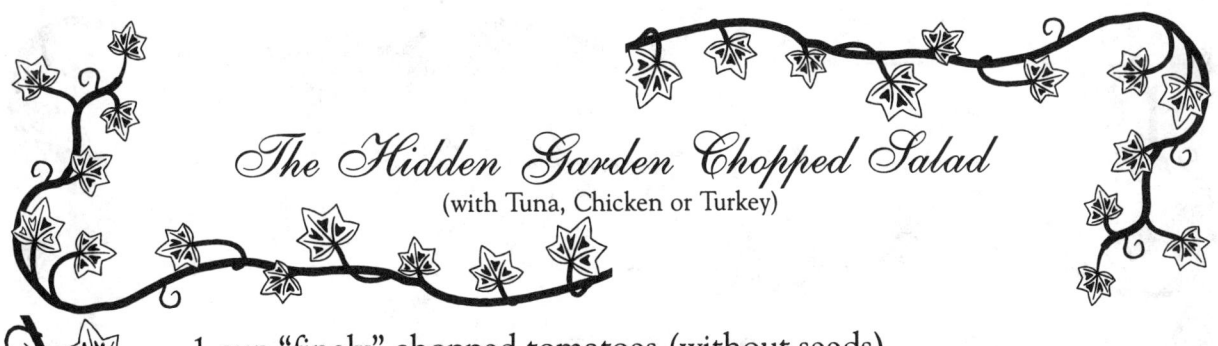

1 cup "finely" chopped tomatoes (without seeds)
1 cup "finely" chopped lettuce
1 hard boiled egg, whites only, chopped
½ "finely" chopped cucumber (without seeds)
½ "finely" chopped red or green pepper
1 tbsp. blue cheese (crumbled)
½ cup chopped grapes
1 scoop tuna (unsalted, packed in water), or
   finely chopped chicken meat or turkey meat.
1 tbsp. fat free mayonnaise
1 tsp. chopped fresh basil

Chop lettuce and cover the salad plate. Clockwise add chopped cucumber, chopped grapes, 1 tablespoon blue cheese. Then carefully arrange one boiled egg whites

Mix tuna, chicken or turkey in a bowl with 1 tablespoon mayonnaise, freshly chopped sweet basil and blend well. Add to a salad plate.

Arrange the chopped tomatoes in the center, forming a mountain. Garnish with sprigs of parsley.

Serve with cucumber dill dressing on the side.

Makes one or two salad platters.

Nola's Note: The secret here is to "finely" chop all ingredients and to arrange the plate artfully!

Mint Cucumber Salad

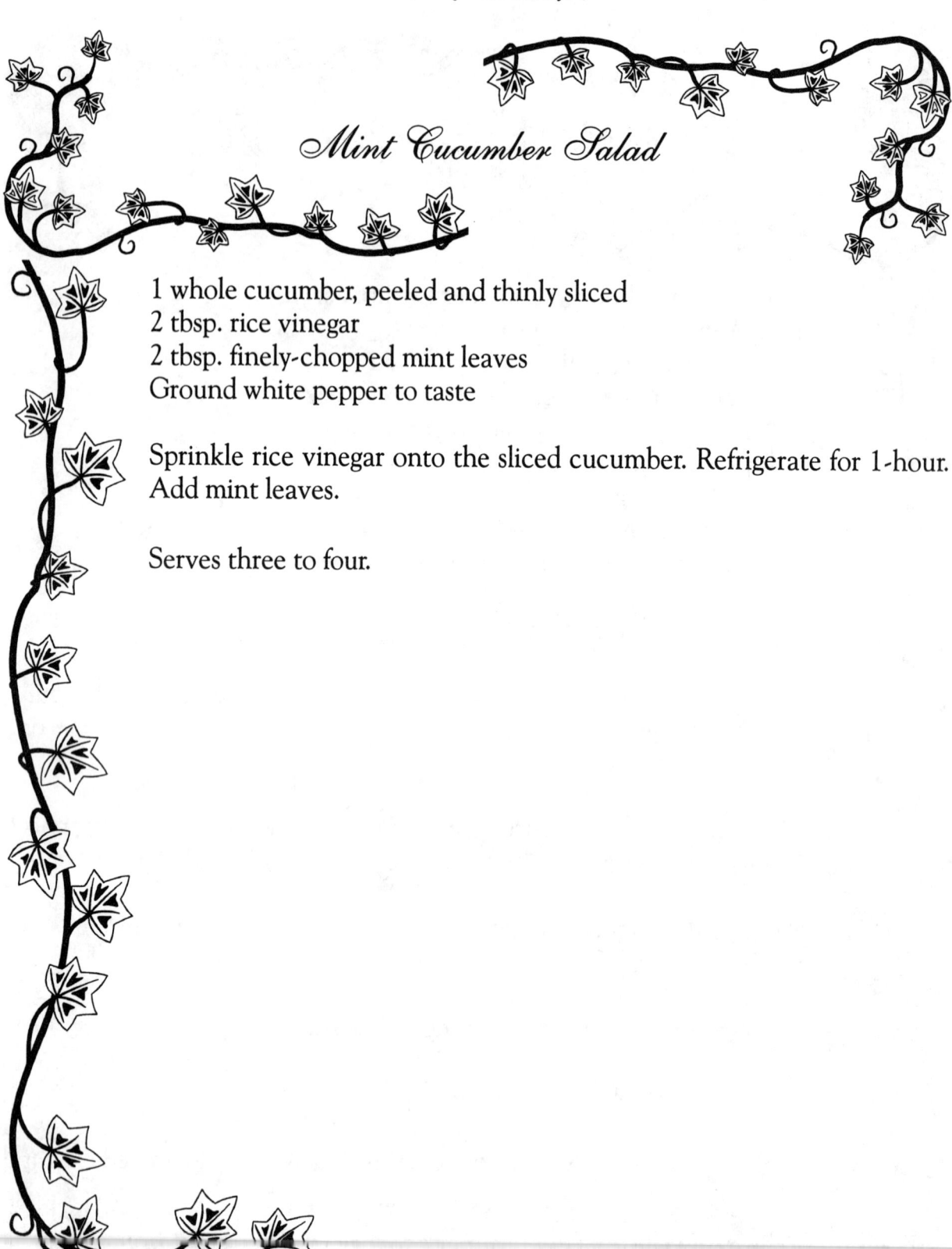

1 whole cucumber, peeled and thinly sliced
2 tbsp. rice vinegar
2 tbsp. finely-chopped mint leaves
Ground white pepper to taste

Sprinkle rice vinegar onto the sliced cucumber. Refrigerate for 1-hour. Add mint leaves.

Serves three to four.

The Hidden Garden Cookbook

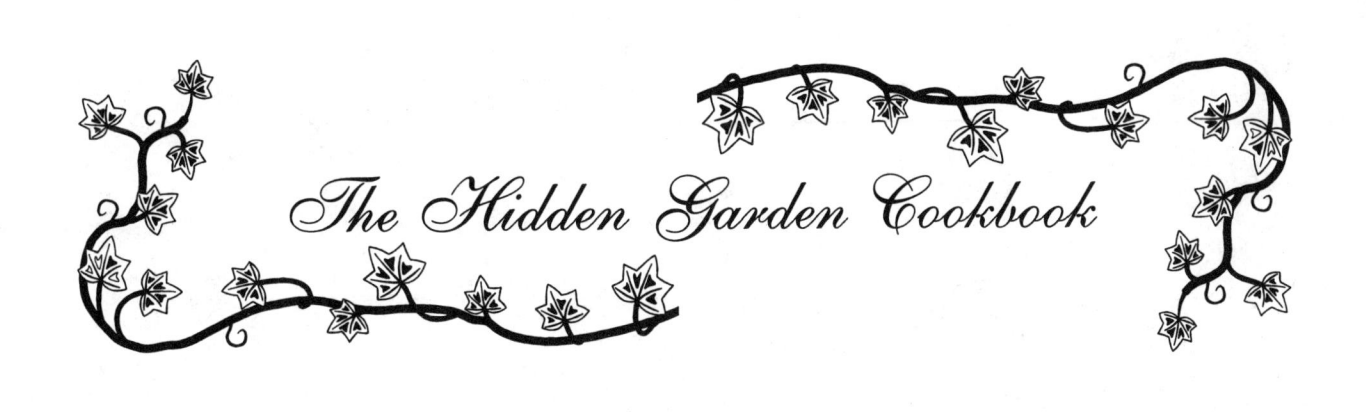

Soups

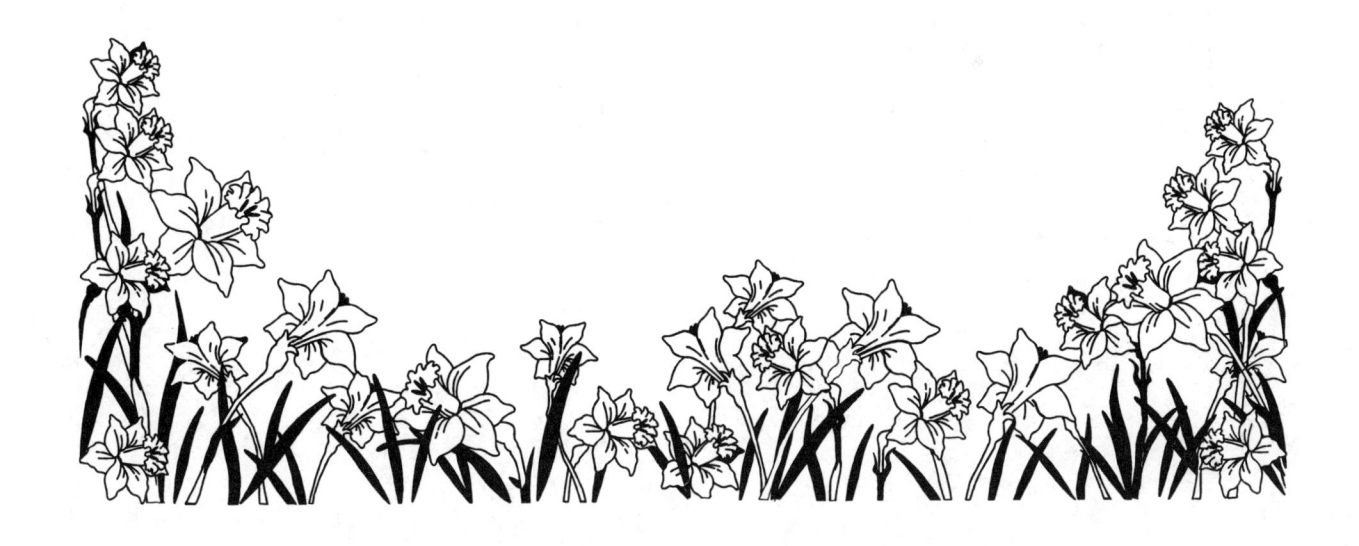

The Hidden Garden Homemade Chicken Soup

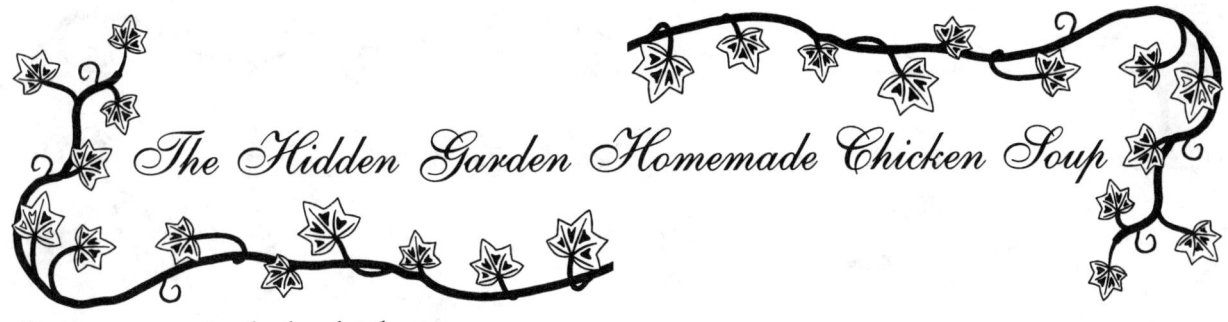

2 whole chickens
1 bunch of parsley
1 dozen big carrots (scrubbed)
1 whole celery cluster (stalks and leaves)
4 cups sliced leek (white part only)

Combine all ingredients in a heavy soup pot. Add enough water to cover. Bring to a boil then reduce heat. Cover and simmer until water is 2/3 of the pot and all ingredients, especially the chicken, are tender. Uncover and let cool.

Strain the soup, removing all solid ingredients. Cover with plastic wrap and refrigerate overnight. Scrape off the solidified fat. Package the broth into containers for freezing.

Serve pure or you may add angel's hair fresh pasta noodles or cooked rice.

Serve warm with sprig of parsley and choice of soft crackers.

Nola's Note: This wonderful chicken soup recipe is used throughout our cookbook and is referred to as Chicken Broth*.

Country Inn Potato Leek Soup

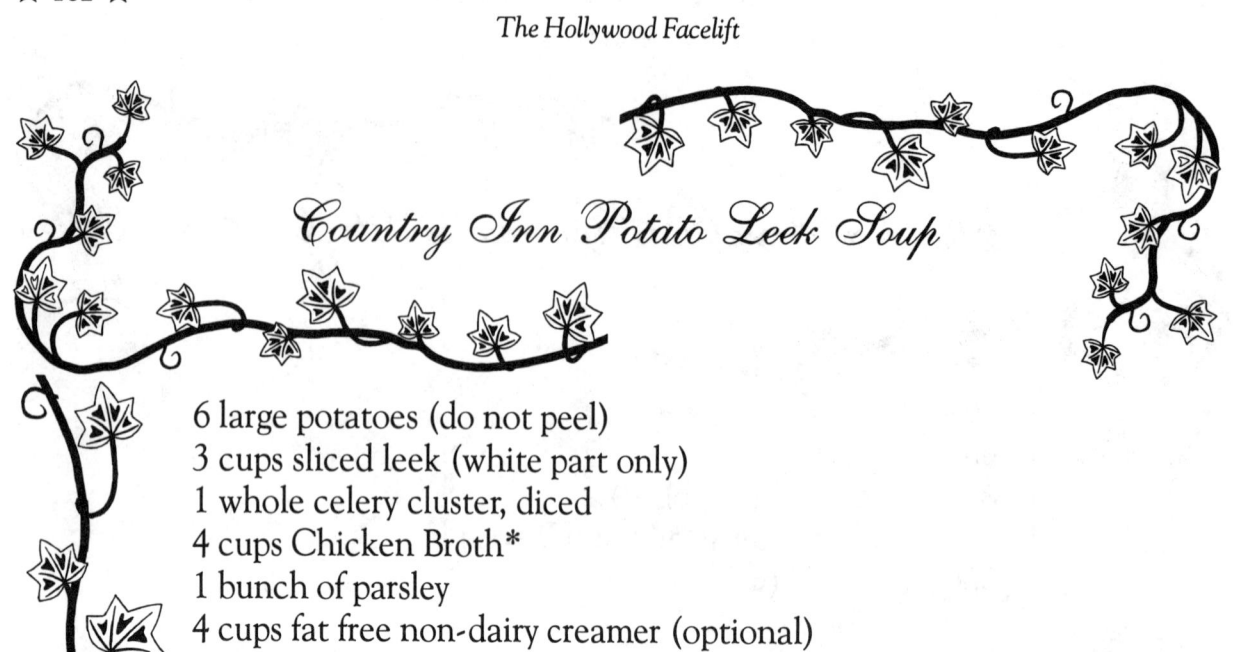

6 large potatoes (do not peel)
3 cups sliced leek (white part only)
1 whole celery cluster, diced
4 cups Chicken Broth*
1 bunch of parsley
4 cups fat free non-dairy creamer (optional)

Dice potatoes. Combine leek, celery, parsley and potatoes in a heavy soup pot. Add water to cover and bring to a boil. Cook until potatoes are soft. Add Chicken Broth*. Simmer 10-minutes. Let cool for an hour. Puree potato/liquid mixture in blender until smooth. Adjust seasoning with dash of pepper. Add non-dairy creamer. Stir. Heat before serving.

Serves six.

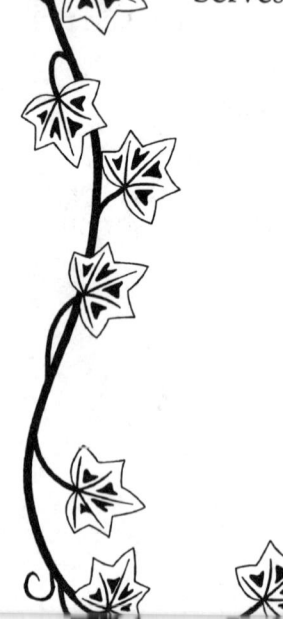

Bay Shrimp Bisque

2 pounds baby Bay Shrimp
6 big carrots chopped
3 cups sliced leek (white part only)
1 cup chopped scallions
4 tblsp. olive oil or vegetable oil
White ground pepper
6 cups Chicken Broth*
2 cups fat free non-dairy creamer

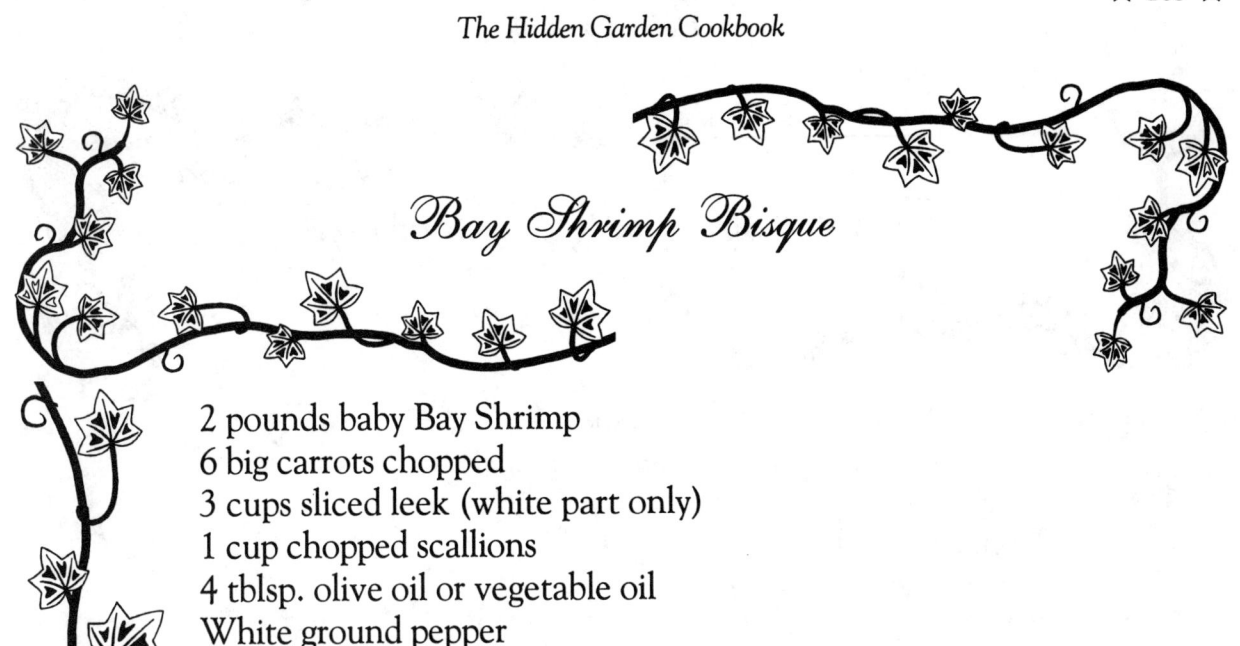

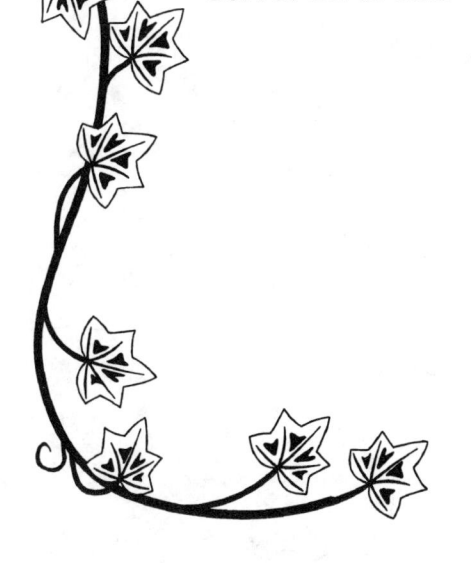

Sauté shrimp in olive oil over medium heat. Add carrots, leek and scallions. Cook for 2 minutes. Add Chicken Broth* and simmer 10 minutes. Put white ground pepper to taste. Remove from heat and cool slightly. Puree in blender. Return to pot and add non-dairy creamer. Stir.

Heat before serving. You may top with parmesan cheese or chopped parsley.

Serves six to ten.

Fresh Tomato Mushroom Bisque

3 cups chopped fresh mushrooms
4 cups fresh tomatoes (pureed, no seeds)
3 tsp. olive or vegetable oil
2 tsp. dill weed
1 tblsp. chopped parsley
½ tsp. ground white pepper
1 cup light sour cream or non-fat yogurt
1 cup fat free non-dairy creamer

Sauté mushrooms in oil until tender. Add tomato puree, dill weed, chopped parsley and stir constantly over medium heat. Simmer for 10 minutes. Reduce heat to low, add sour cream and white pepper to taste. Pour into a heavy pot and mix non-dairy creamer. Stir until well blended. Heat before serving.

Garnish with chopped chives or sprigs of parsley.

Serves four.

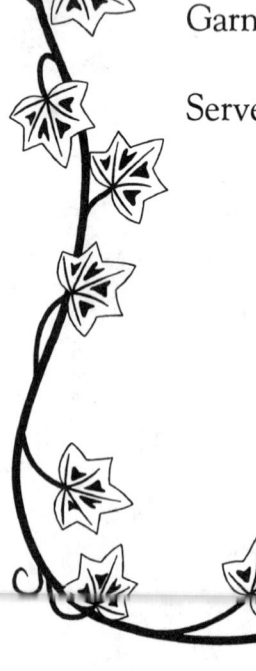

The Hidden Garden Homemade Carrot Soup

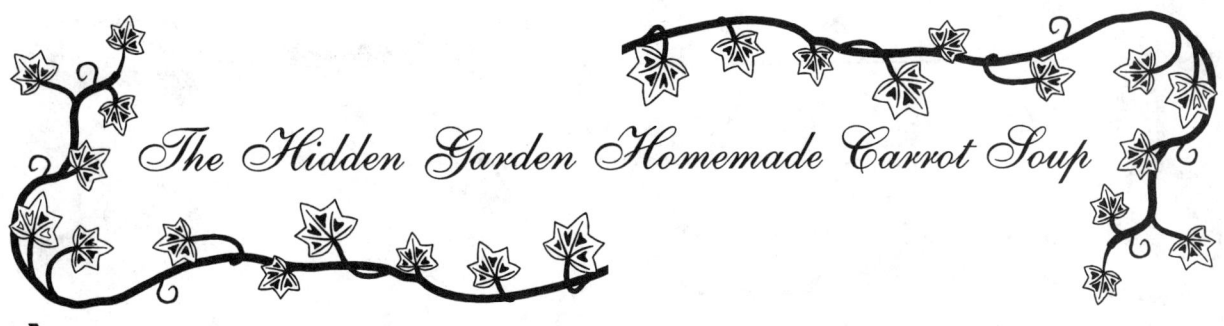

2 dozen big Carrots (scrubbed)
1 whole celery cluster
2 bunches of parsley
3 cups slices leek (white part only)
1 tsp. fennel seed
6 cups Chicken Broth*
1 tsp. ground white pepper

Combine all ingredients except Chicken Broth* in a heavy soup pot. Add enough water to cover. Bring to a boil, then simmer until carrots are tender. Remove from heat and let stand for at least one hour. Strain the soup reserving the liquid. Set aside carrots. Transfer cooked carrots to food blender, adding the reserved cooking liquid as needed. Puree until smooth.

Pour the pureed carrots into a clean pot and add the Chicken Broth. Simmer 10 minutes over medium heat. Season with ground white pepper to taste.

If you want a creamier flavor, add 2 cups non-dairy creamer.

Serves eight to ten.

Broccoli Soup

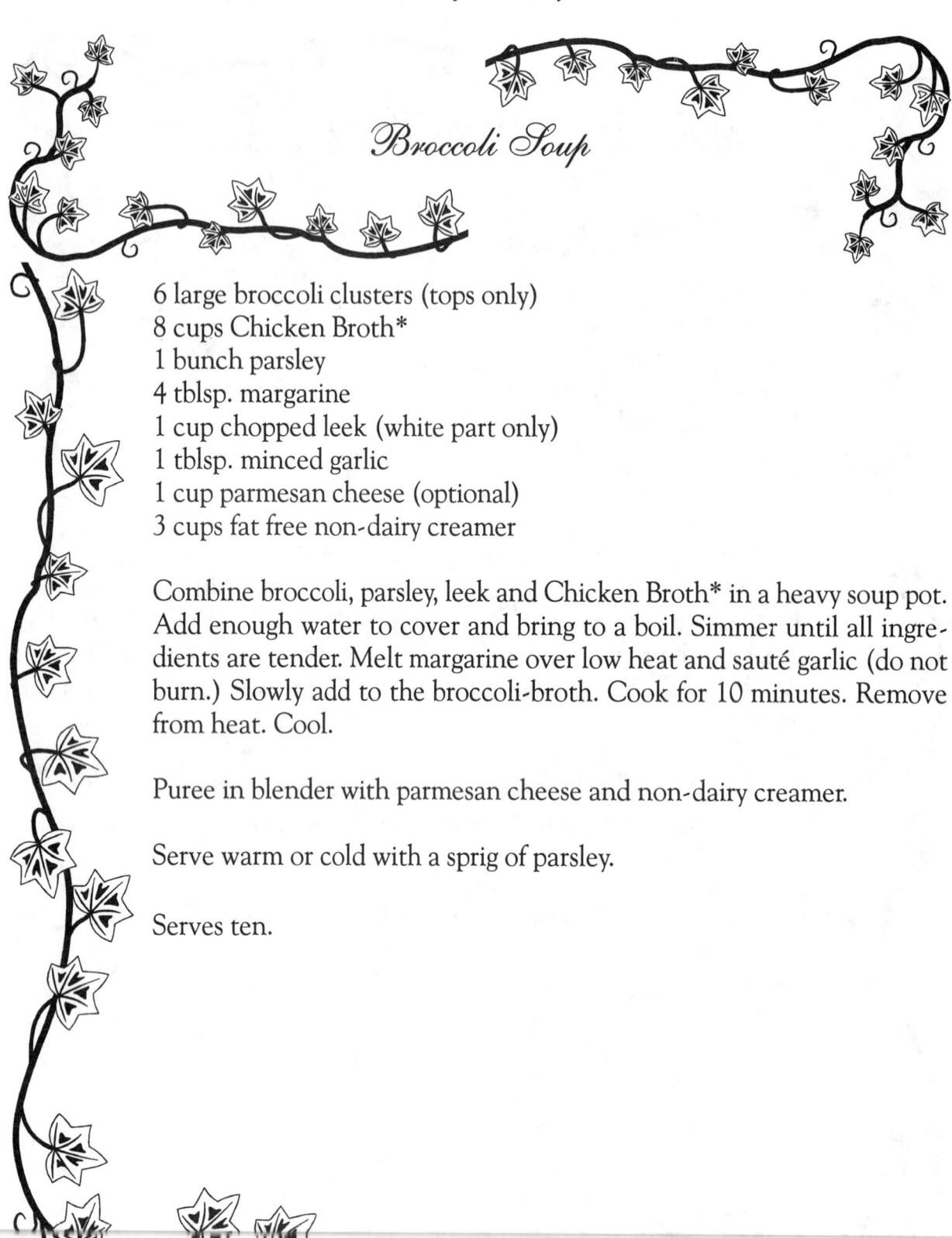

6 large broccoli clusters (tops only)
8 cups Chicken Broth*
1 bunch parsley
4 tblsp. margarine
1 cup chopped leek (white part only)
1 tblsp. minced garlic
1 cup parmesan cheese (optional)
3 cups fat free non-dairy creamer

Combine broccoli, parsley, leek and Chicken Broth* in a heavy soup pot. Add enough water to cover and bring to a boil. Simmer until all ingredients are tender. Melt margarine over low heat and sauté garlic (do not burn.) Slowly add to the broccoli-broth. Cook for 10 minutes. Remove from heat. Cool.

Puree in blender with parmesan cheese and non-dairy creamer.

Serve warm or cold with a sprig of parsley.

Serves ten.

Garden Fresh Chunky Vegetable Soup

8 large potatoes (do not peel)
8 large carrots (scrubbed)
8 cups Chicken Broth*
2 packs frozen corn kernels
1 cup chopped parsley
1 cup chopped leek (white part only)
1 cluster celery, chopped
4 tblsp. thyme
2 tsp. ground white pepper (optional)

Cook potatoes and carrots in a heavy soup pot with Chicken Broth* and enough water to cover. Let boil then simmer until tender. Add leeks, celery, corn, parsley and thyme. Stir well, breaking up the carrots and potatoes. Simmer for 30 minutes.

Season with ground white pepper.

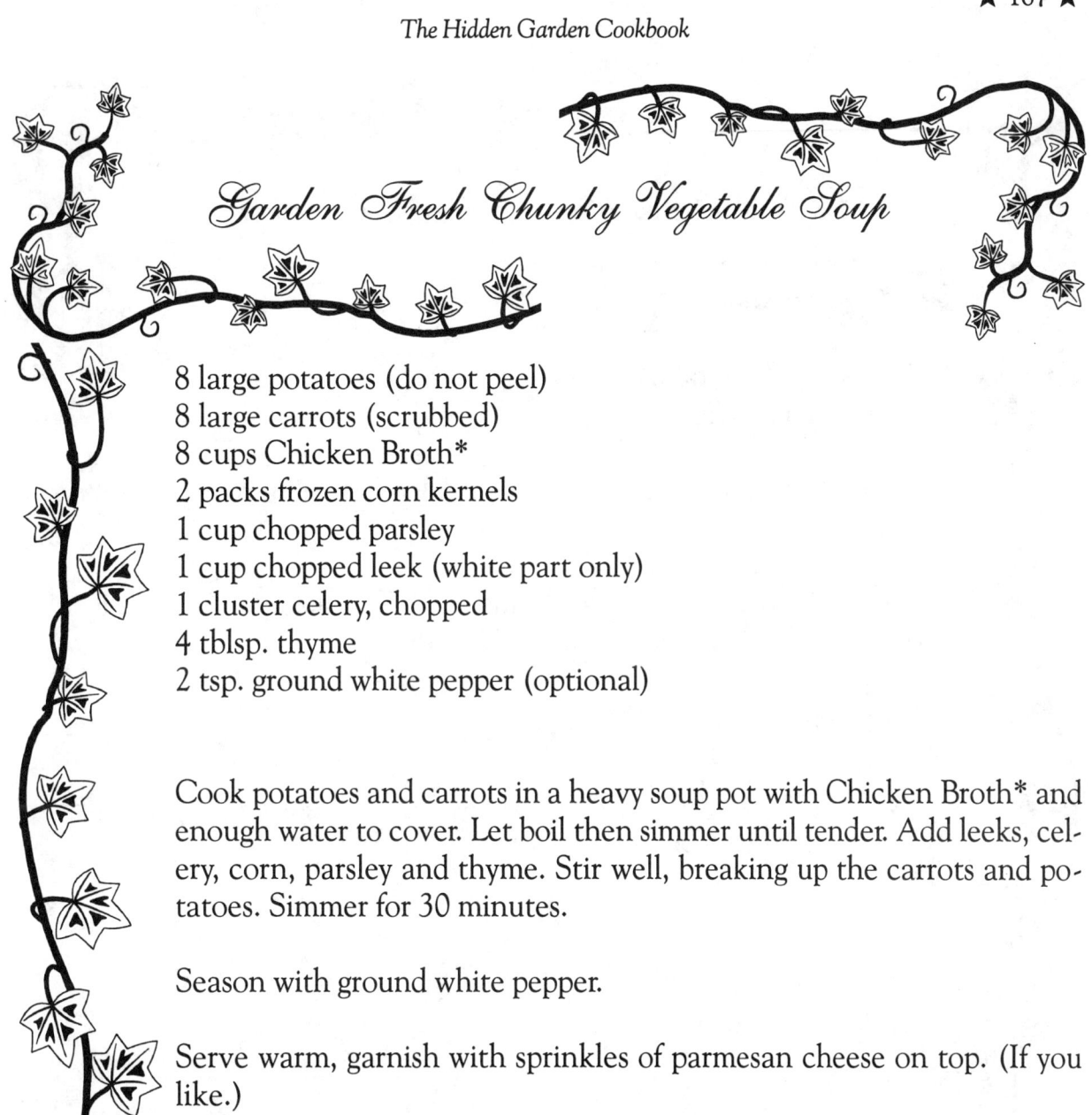

Serve warm, garnish with sprinkles of parmesan cheese on top. (If you like.)

Nola's Note: It's a wonderful winter soup left chunky! May be pureed in the blender for soft-diet patients.

P.S. This is not just any vegetable soup. This is incredible!

Chilled Cantaloupe-Pineapple Soup

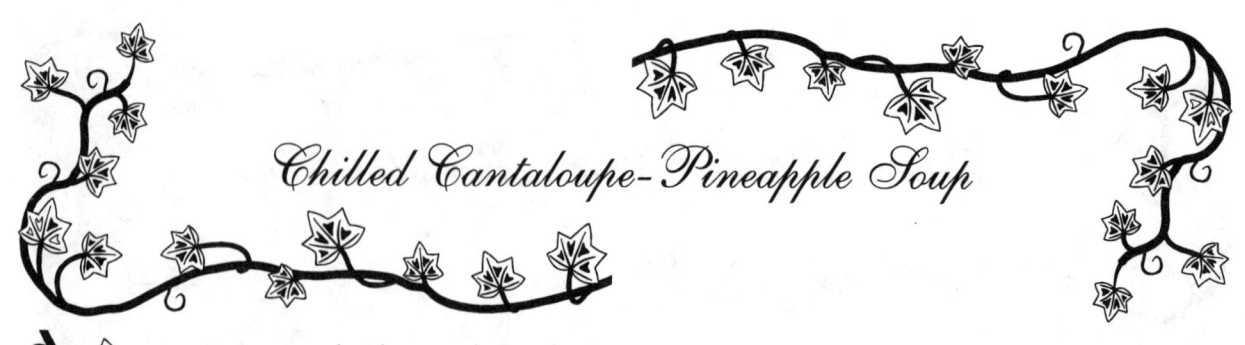

2 cups cubed cantaloupe fruit
½ cup chopped fresh pineapple

Puree cantaloupe fruit in a blender. Add chopped pineapple and puree until smooth.

Serve cold in a chilled bowl. Garnish with thin sliver lemon slice floating on top with a mint leaf.

Serves one.

The Hidden Garden Cookbook

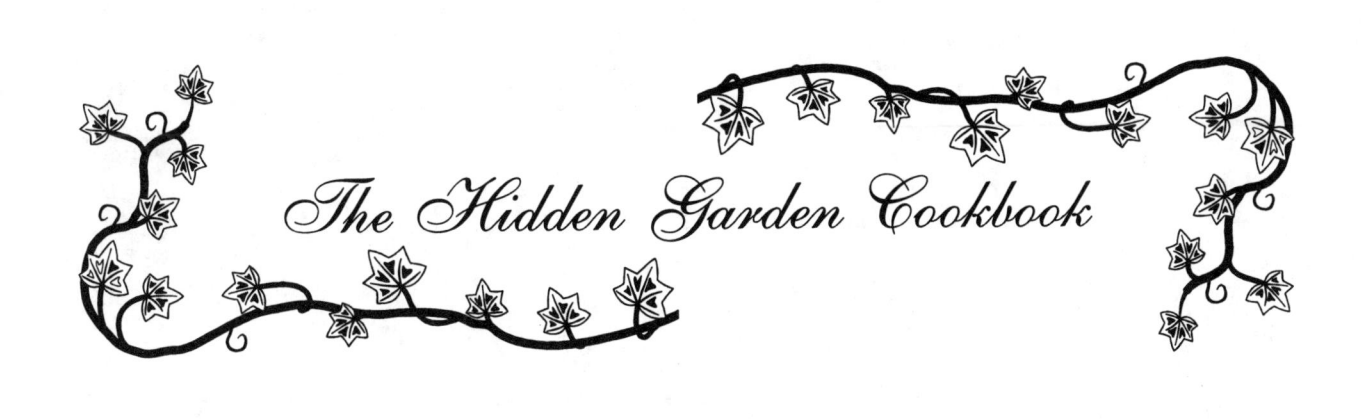

Omelet

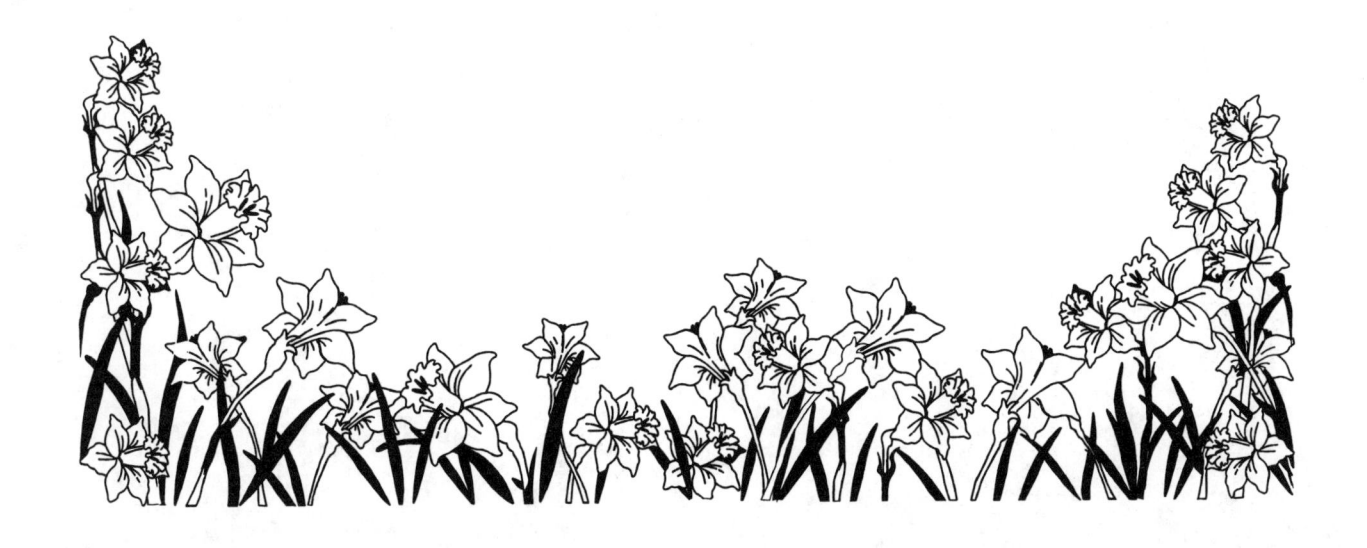

Avocado and Cream Omelette

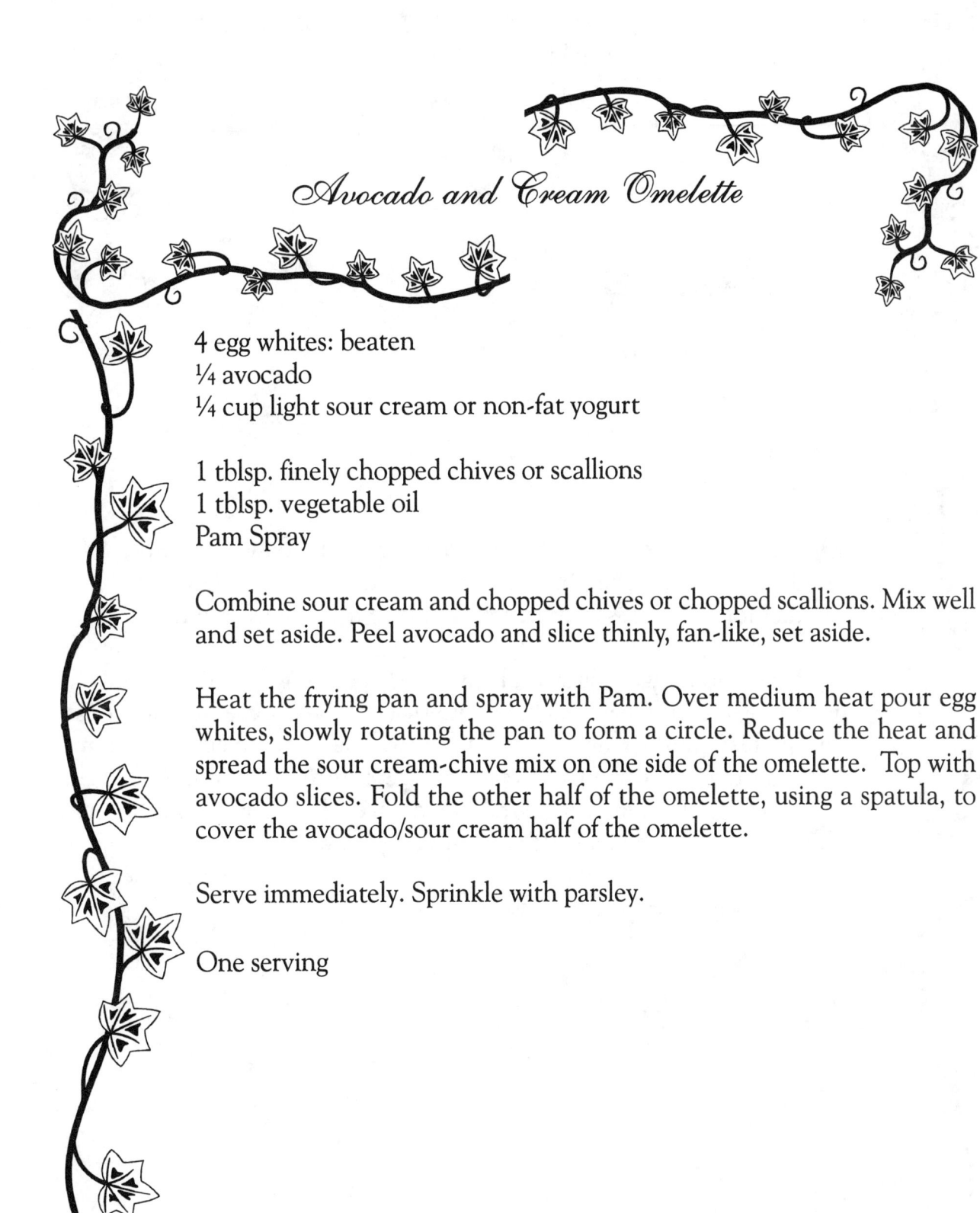

4 egg whites: beaten
¼ avocado
¼ cup light sour cream or non-fat yogurt

1 tblsp. finely chopped chives or scallions
1 tblsp. vegetable oil
Pam Spray

Combine sour cream and chopped chives or chopped scallions. Mix well and set aside. Peel avocado and slice thinly, fan-like, set aside.

Heat the frying pan and spray with Pam. Over medium heat pour egg whites, slowly rotating the pan to form a circle. Reduce the heat and spread the sour cream-chive mix on one side of the omelette. Top with avocado slices. Fold the other half of the omelette, using a spatula, to cover the avocado/sour cream half of the omelette.

Serve immediately. Sprinkle with parsley.

One serving

Mushroom Omelette

4 egg whites: beaten
1 cup thinly sliced mushrooms
1 tsp. chives
1 tblsp. vegetable oil
Pam Spray

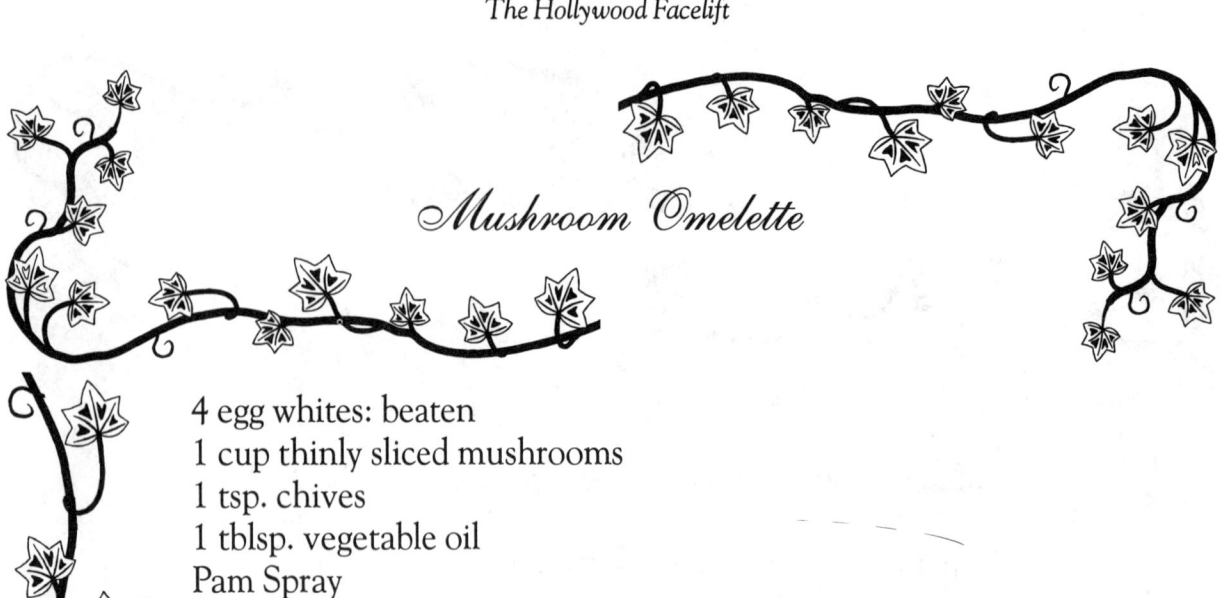

Heat one tablespoon vegetable oil in a sauté pan. Sauté mushrooms for 5-minutes over medium heat. Season with dash of pepper. Cover and let simmer for 2-minutes or until soft. Remove from heat. Strain.

Spray a heated frying pan with Pam. Slowly pour into pan the beaten egg whites. Rotate the pan. Let cook for 30-seconds on a medium-low heat. Put sautéed mushrooms on one half side of the egg omelette. Cover and reduce heat. Continue to cook for 30-seconds to one-minute. Fold the other half of omelette using a spatula to cover the side with mushrooms. Transfer to a lunch plate and serve immediately.

Sprinkle with chopped parsley.

Serves one

Spinach Omelette

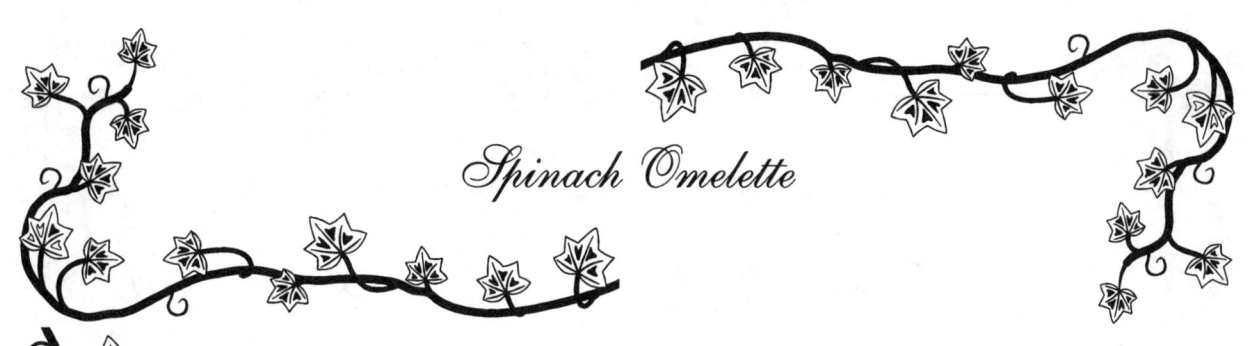

4 egg whites: beaten
2 cups clean & dry spinach leaves
1 tblsp. pine nuts
1 tblsp. vegetable oil
Pam Spray
1 clove garlic: chopped

Put spinach and pine nuts in food processor and chop finely. Sauté garlic in heated skillet with 1 tblsp. vegetable oil. Add chopped spinach and pine nuts. Sauté for 1-minute covered. Remove from heat.

Use Pam Spray in a pan. Pour beaten egg whites while rotating the pan to form a circle. Let cook for at least 30-seconds on a medium-low heat. Spread cooked spinach on one side or half omelette. Cover and reduce heat. Let cook for 30-seconds to one minute. Fold the other half of the omelette, using a spatula, to cover the side with the spinach mixture.

Serve warm on a lunch plate with Italian parsley and slices of tomato.

Serves one.

Goat Cheese Omelette

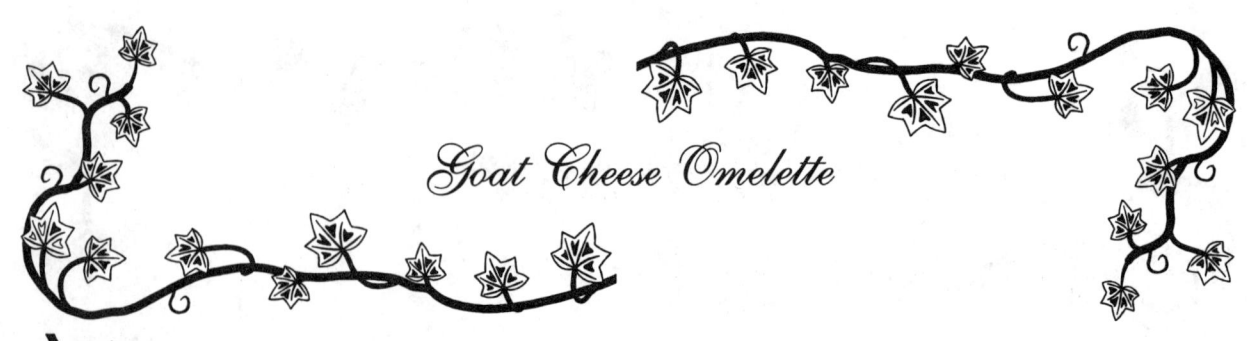

4 egg whites: beaten
4 thin slices of goat cheese
1 tsp. chopped scallions
Pam Spray

Spray frying pan with Pam. Slowly pour the well-beaten egg whites while rotating the pan to form a circle. Cover and let cook for at least 30-seconds. Spread the thin slices of cheese and chopped scallions on one side of the omelette. Cover and continue to cook over low heat for 30-seconds to 1-minute. Fold the other side of omelette, using a spatula, to cover the side with cheese as it starts to melt.

Serve immediately with sprigs of parsley and orange wedges.

Serves one.

The Hidden Garden Cookbook

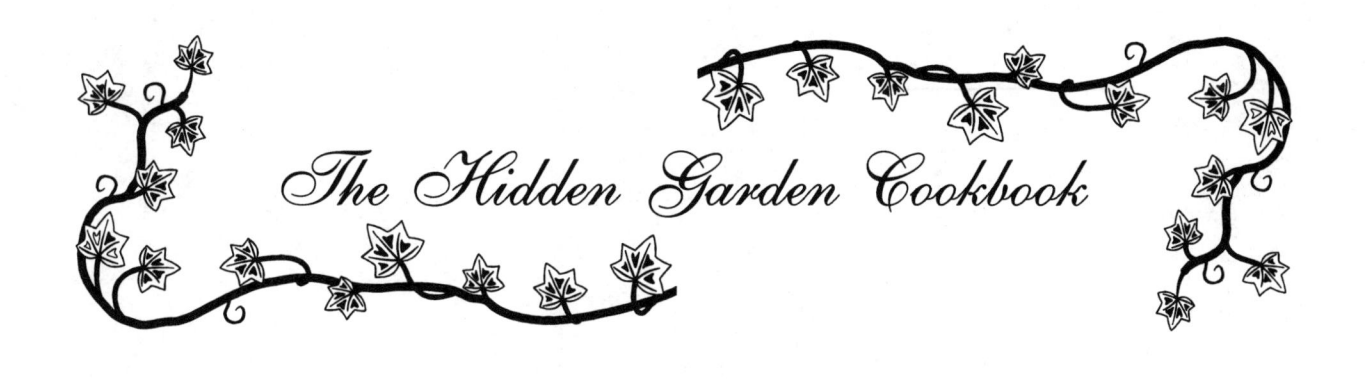

Fish

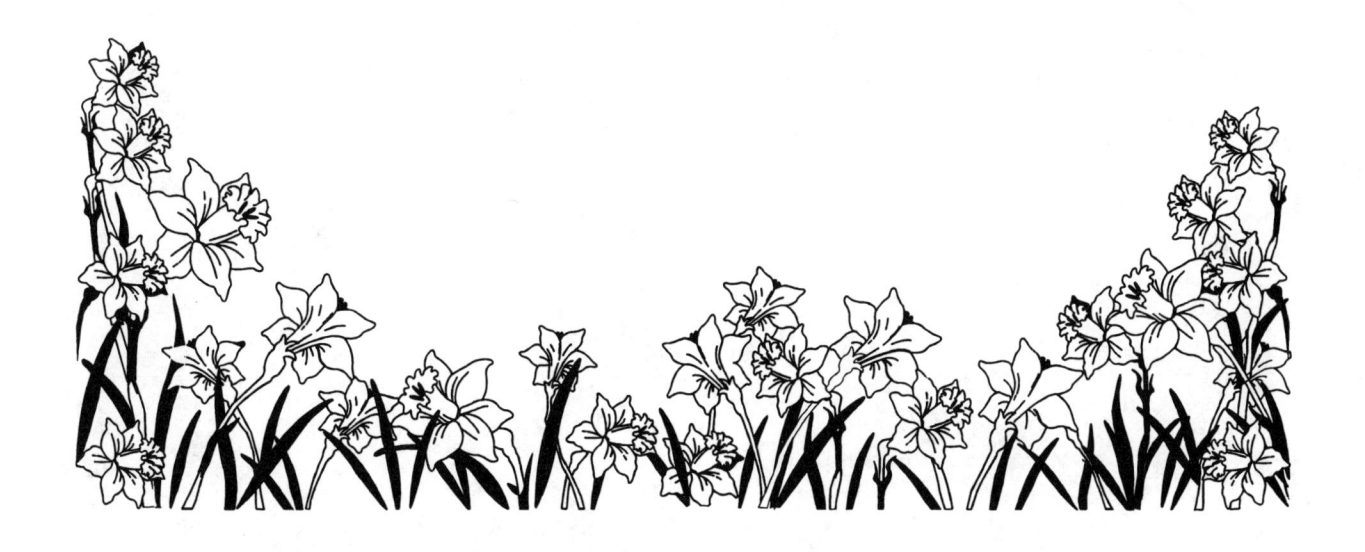

Broiled Chilean Sea Bass

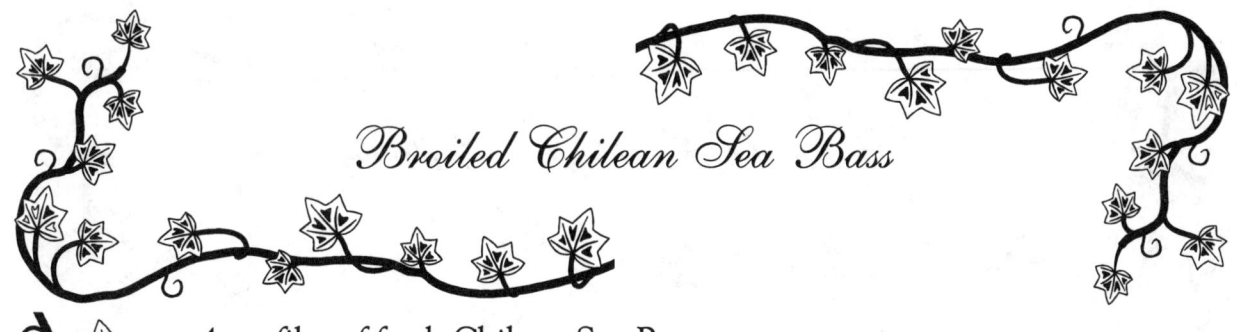

4 oz. filet of fresh Chilean Sea Bass
½ tsp. dill weed
1 tsp. lemon juice

Preheat the oven to 400°. Place filet on a clean non-stick baking dish. Mix dill weed, and lemon juice. Brush each piece of Sea Bass generously with dill-lemon mixture.

Broil each piece of Sea Bass 6 to 10-minutes depending on the thickness of the fish.

Garnish with slices of tomato or chopped tomato salad and Italian parsley.

Serves one.

Poached Norwegian Salmon

4 oz. filet of fresh Norwegian Salmon
½ tsp. dill weed
Lemon wedges for garnishing
Italian parsley

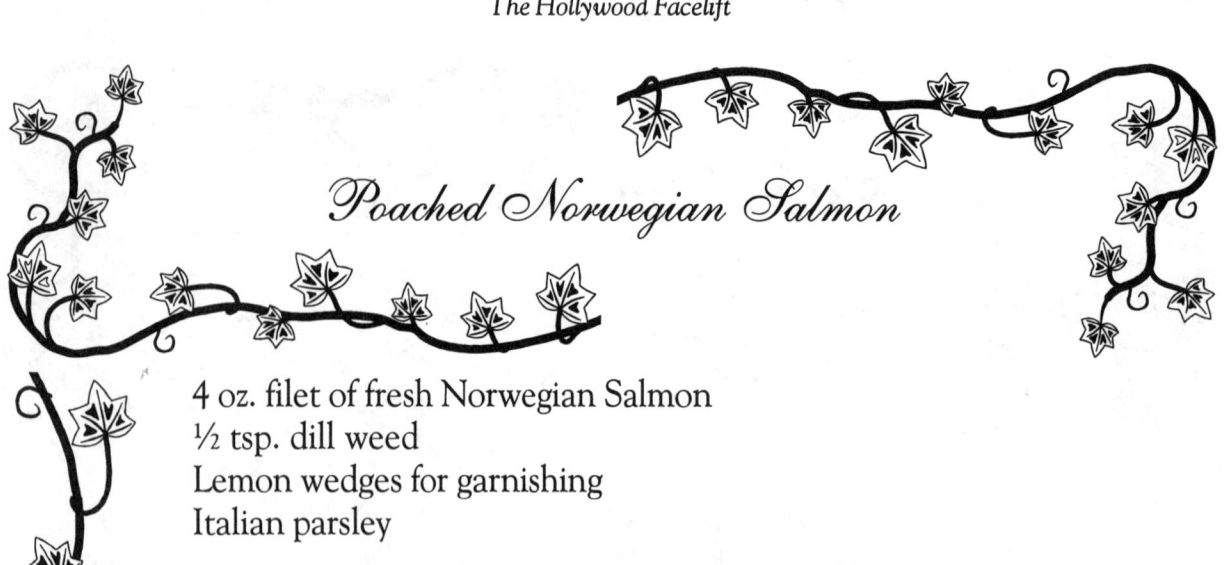

Preheat the over to 400°F. Place the salmon on a sheet of aluminum foil. Fold up edges and seal tight.

Bake for 6 to 10-minutes depending on thickness. Serve at once. Sprinkle with dill weed and garnish with Italian parsley and lemon wedges.

Serves one.

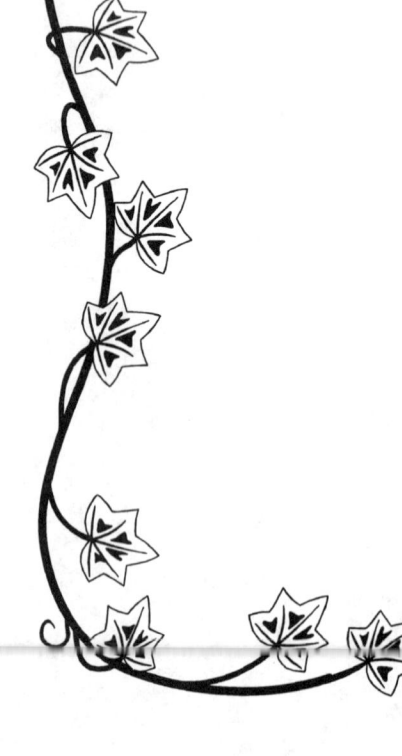

Bay Scallops

2 pounds Bay Scallops
1 garlic clove minced
2 tblsp. virgin olive oil
White pepper to taste
Chopped fresh basil

In a large sauté pan or skillet, heat olive oil. Sauté scallops for 2-minutes, add minced garlic, and sauté altogether continuously for 3-minutes. Season with chopped basil and white ground pepper to taste.

Garnish with slices of tomato, orange wedges and sprigs of parsley.

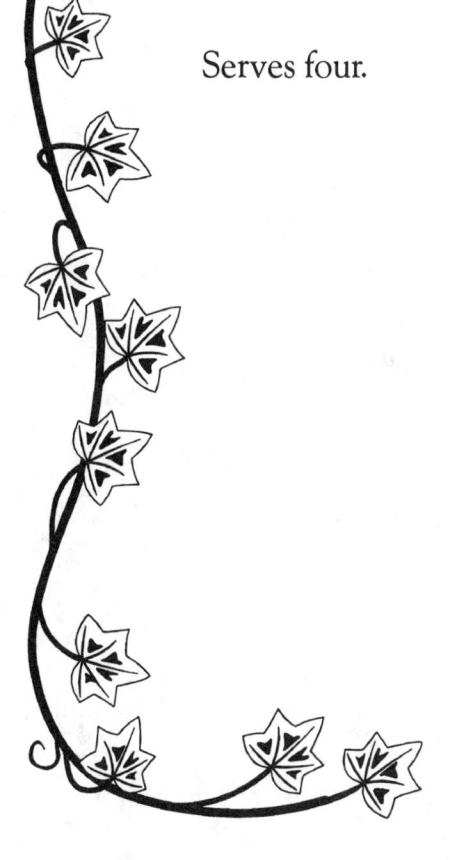

Serves four.

Nola's Scampi and Herbs

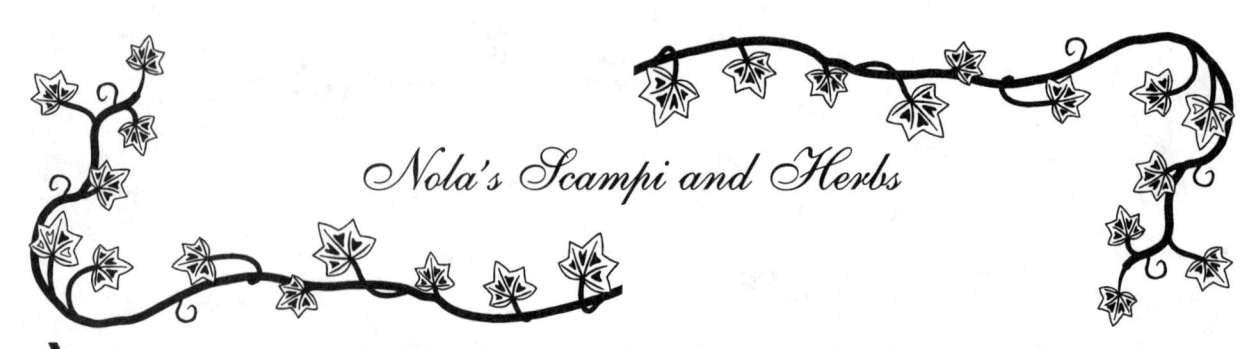

12-16 Jumbo Scampi: butterflied, shells and tails left intact
3 tblsp. virgin olive oil
1 tblsp. fresh basil, chopped
1½ tblsp. crushed red pepper
½ tblsp. garlic minced
2 tblsp. fresh parsley, chopped
2 tblsp. grated lemon peel

Heat 3 tblsp. olive oil in a large skillet over medium heat. Sauté garlic. Add Scampi shell side up and sauté about 2-minutes. Cover and let steam until cooked (2-4 minutes). Sprinkle with herbs. Season to taste.

Serve immediately with Pasta with Pesto.

Serves four.

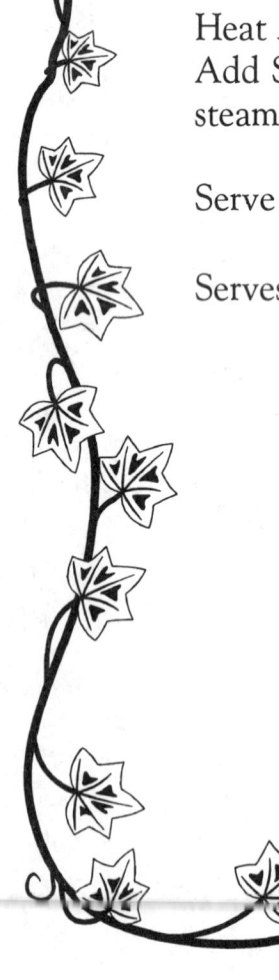

The Hidden Garden Cookbook

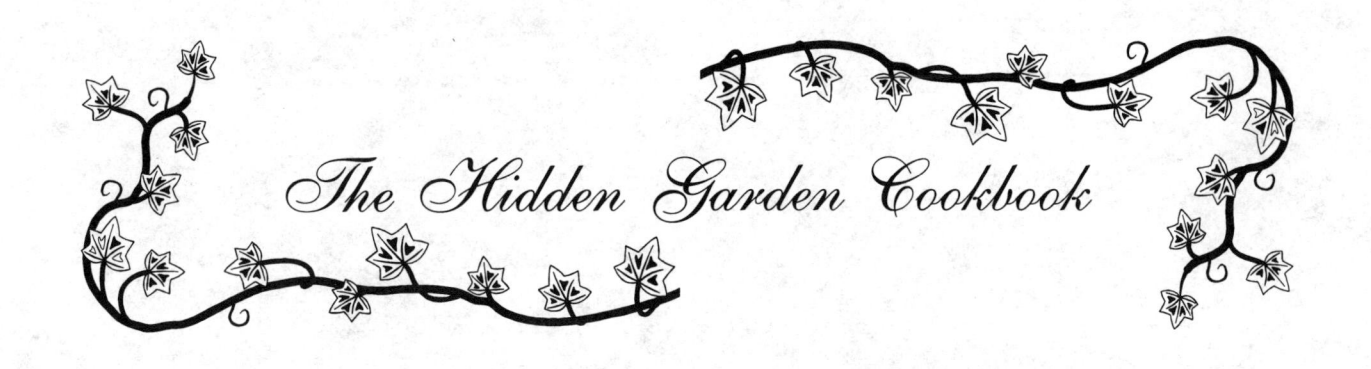

Chicken

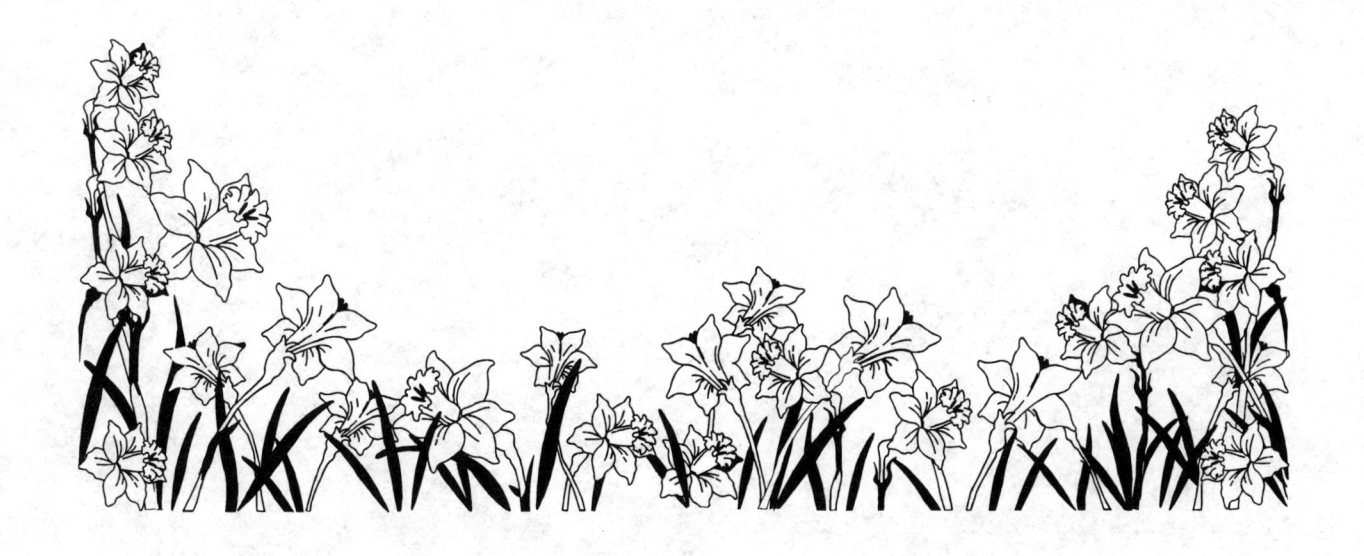

Chicken Picatta with Fresh Garden Herbs

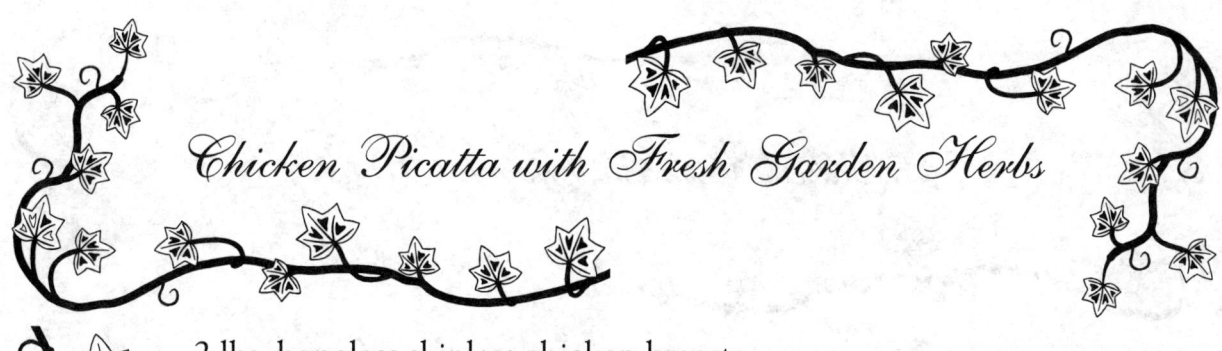

2 lbs. boneless skinless chicken breasts
4 cups plain breadcrumbs
1½ cups finely-chopped Italian parsley
1 cup finely-chopped fresh basil leaves
1 tblsp. oregano
3 egg whites
Vegetable oil

Take each chicken breast and pound between sheets of plastic wrap or inside a plastic baggie. Dip pounded chicken breast in well beaten egg whites.

Meanwhile, mix breadcrumbs, chopped parsley, basil leaves and oregano. Place breadcrumbs mixture in a huge plate and press egg-dipped chicken breast into the breadcrumbs. Shake to remove excess breadcrumbs and sauté in vegetable oil over medium heat until brown. Add 1-2 tablespoons of water and cover. Steam until dry and tender.

Serve warm or cold, sliced or whole breast with a sprig of parsley and lemon wedges.

Serves six to seven.

Nola's Note: Prepared seasoned bread crumbs are too salty!

Baked Cornish Game Hens

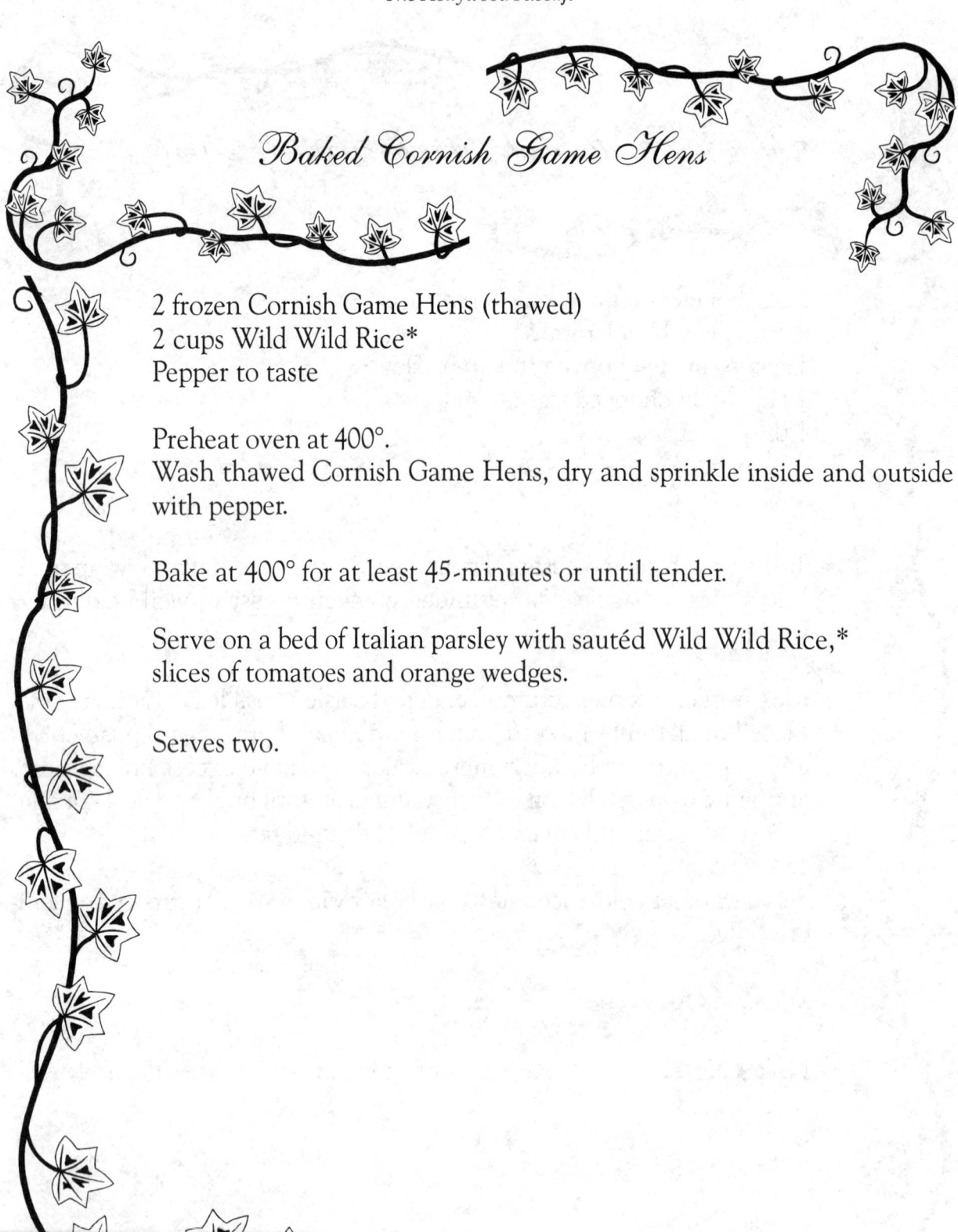

2 frozen Cornish Game Hens (thawed)
2 cups Wild Wild Rice*
Pepper to taste

Preheat oven at 400°.
Wash thawed Cornish Game Hens, dry and sprinkle inside and outside with pepper.

Bake at 400° for at least 45-minutes or until tender.

Serve on a bed of Italian parsley with sautéd Wild Wild Rice,* slices of tomatoes and orange wedges.

Serves two.

The Hidden Garden Cookbook

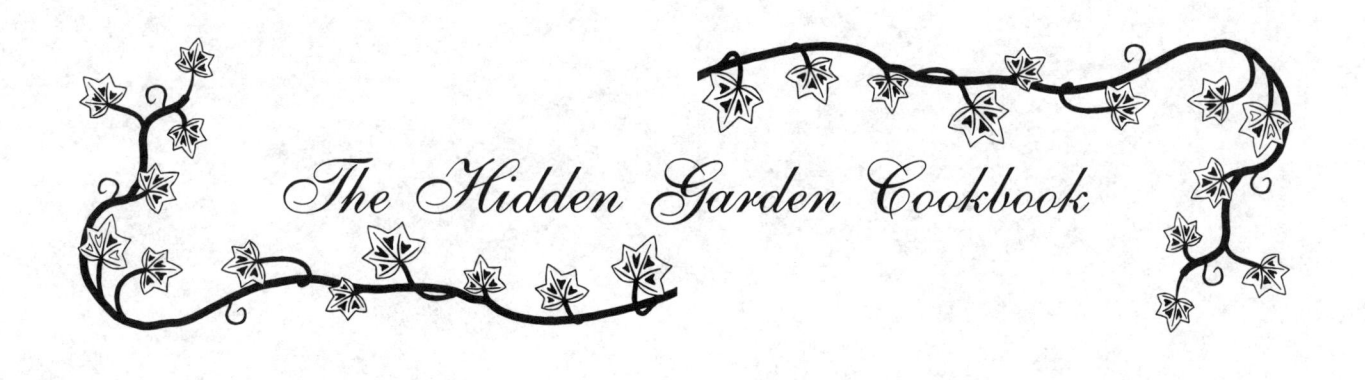

Pasta

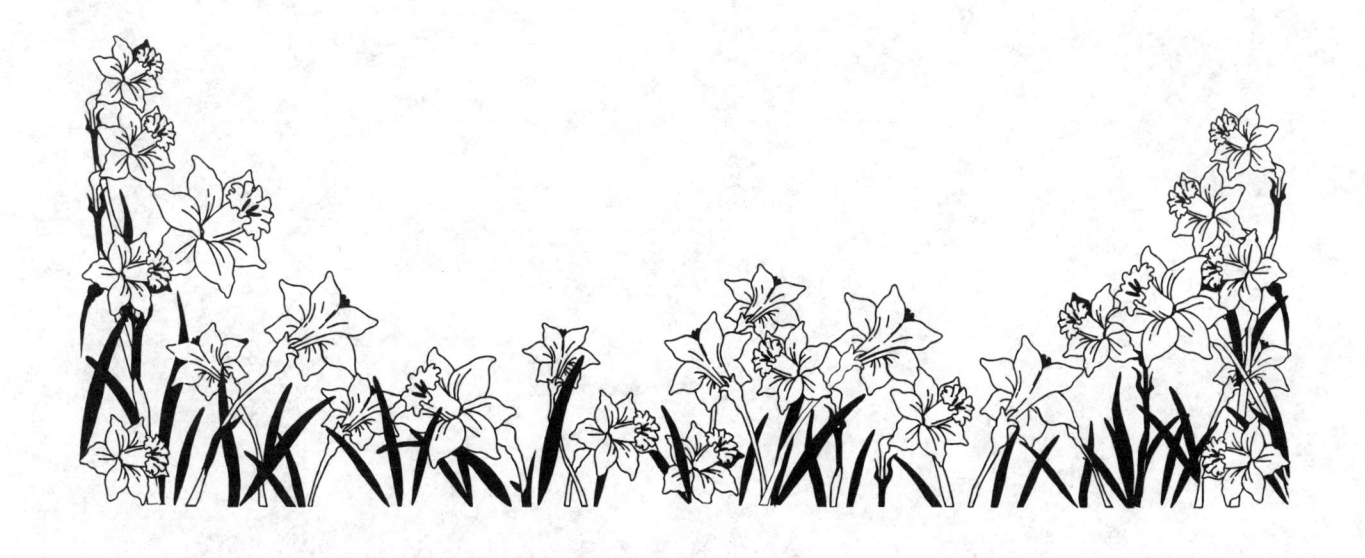

The Hidden Garden Homemade Manicotti

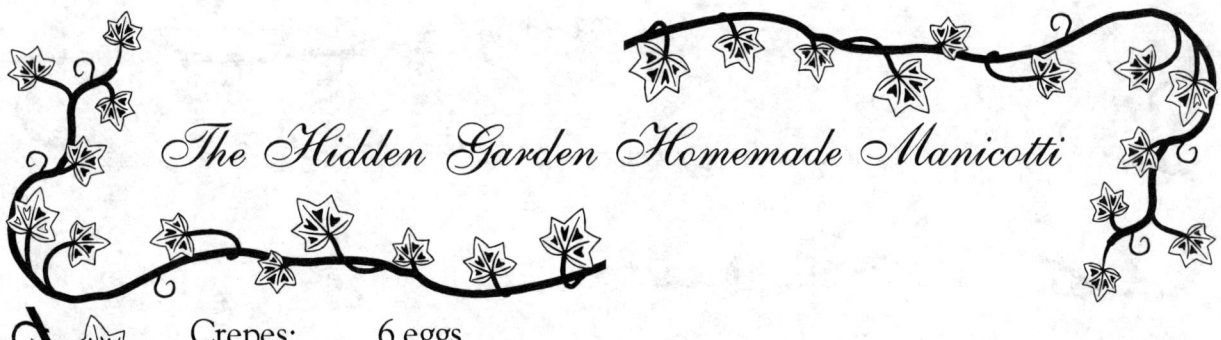

Crepes:
: 6 eggs
: 1½ cups all purpose flour
: 1½ cups water

Filling:
: 32 oz. fat free ricotta cheese
: 1½ cups finely-chopped parsley
: 1 cup shredded parmesan cheese

Sauce:
: 1½ cups prepared chunky tomato sauce (cook's choice)
: ½ cup chopped Italian parsley
: 2 cups chopped tomatoes (without seeds)
: 1 tblsp. chopped fresh basil leaves

Crepes: Combine eggs, flour and water and beat with electric mixer until very smooth. Slowly heat a small skillet. Over low heat pour in 3-4 tablespoons batter, rotating the skillet. Put the cooked crepes on a lined plastic wrap sprayed with Pam to prevent from sticking.

Filling: Put ricotta cheese in a large bowl. Add chopped parsley and parmesan cheese. Blend well using a rubber spatula. Spread about ½ cup filling down the center of each crepe then roll. Place on a non-stick baking pan.

Top with Sauce: Combine tomato sauce, chopped parsley, chopped basil leaves, and stir well until blended. Add 2-cups freshly chopped tomatoes to make it very chunky. Stir well before putting on top of Manicotti. Bake at 375° for 15-minutes.

Garnish with sprigs of parsley and fan slices of Steamed Scallopini squash.*

Makes 16-18 manicotti.

The Hidden Garden Pasta with Pesto

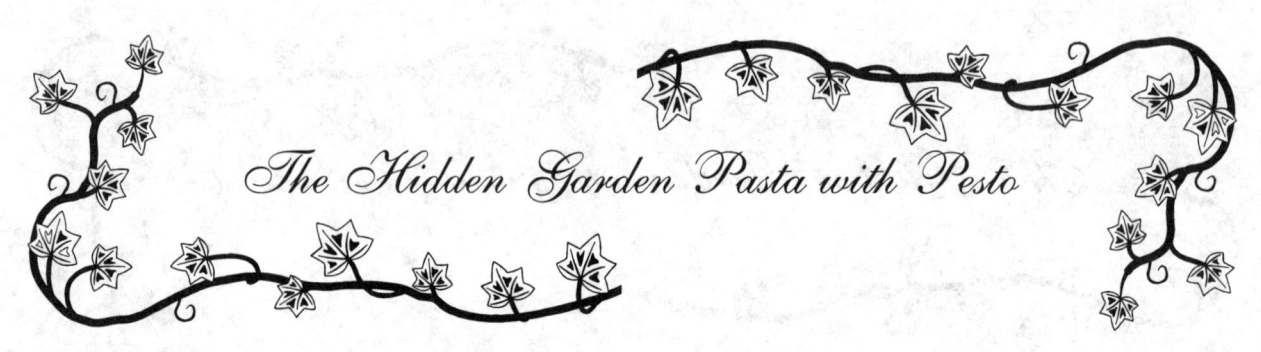

16 oz. fresh linguine
½ cup pine nuts
2 cups fresh basil leaves
½ cup virgin olive oil
2 tblsp. finely chopped garlic
1 cup shredded parmesan cheese

Pesto: Put pine nuts and fresh basil leaves in food processor and chop well. Add olive oil, parmesan cheese, and garlic and blend well until it becomes a sauce. Add additional oil if necessary.

Meanwhile, cook pasta until al dente. Remove from heat and drain well. Rinse in cold water and drain again.

Gradually mix pasta in a large salad bowl, adding the pesto sauce, toss until blended. Or simply serve the pasta on a dinner plate topped with pesto sauce and sprinkled with parmesan cheese.

Garnish with sprigs of Italian parsley.

May be served with Nola's Scampi and Herbs.*

Serve at room temperature.

Serves two to four.

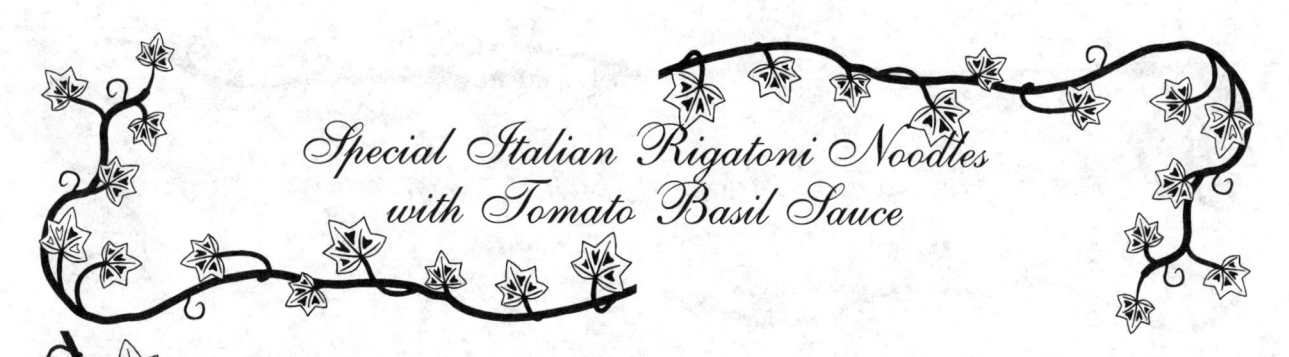

Special Italian Rigatoni Noodles with Tomato Basil Sauce

16 oz. Rigatoni noodles
1 jar prepared tomato sauce (cook's choice)
1 tblsp. virgin olive oil
1 cup finely chopped Italian parsley
2 cups freshly chopped tomatoes (seeds removed)
1 tblsp. garlic, chopped
2 tblsp. finely chopped fresh basil leaves
½ cup shredded parmesan cheese (optional)

Over low heat, sauté garlic in olive oil (do not burn). Add prepared tomato sauce and chopped parsley. Simmer, stirring continuously for 10 minutes. Remove from heat and add 2 cups chopped tomatoes to make sauce chunky. Stir well. Add chopped basil.

Cook Rigatoni noodles in boiling water until tender but still firm to the bite. Transfer the noodles to a bowl of cold water. Drain well.

Arrange Rigatoni noodles in a pasta platter, top with cooked tomato sauce and sprinkle with parsley and parmesan cheese.

Serves two to four.

Grandma Rocco's Pasta Primavera

2 cups broccoli flowers (steamed)
3 cups mushrooms, sliced and sautéed in margarine
2 cups tomatoes, seeds removed, chopped
16 oz. cooked fresh pasta/linguine
½ cup parmesan cheese, roughly grated

Sauce:
4 oz. margarine
4 oz. whipped light cream cheese
4 oz. fat free non-dairy creamer

Slowly melt margarine over low heat, gradually add cream cheese while stirring constantly. Add non-dairy creamer, continue stirring.

Gradually add cooked pasta, a little at a time. Toss gently to coat until all pasta is beautifully coated with sauce.

Serve on an oval-shape pasta plate, topped with parmesan cheese. Arrange on top of pasta ribbons of sautéed mushrooms, steamed broccoli, and chopped tomatoes.

Garnish with Italian parsley.

Serves two to four.

The Hidden Garden Cookbook

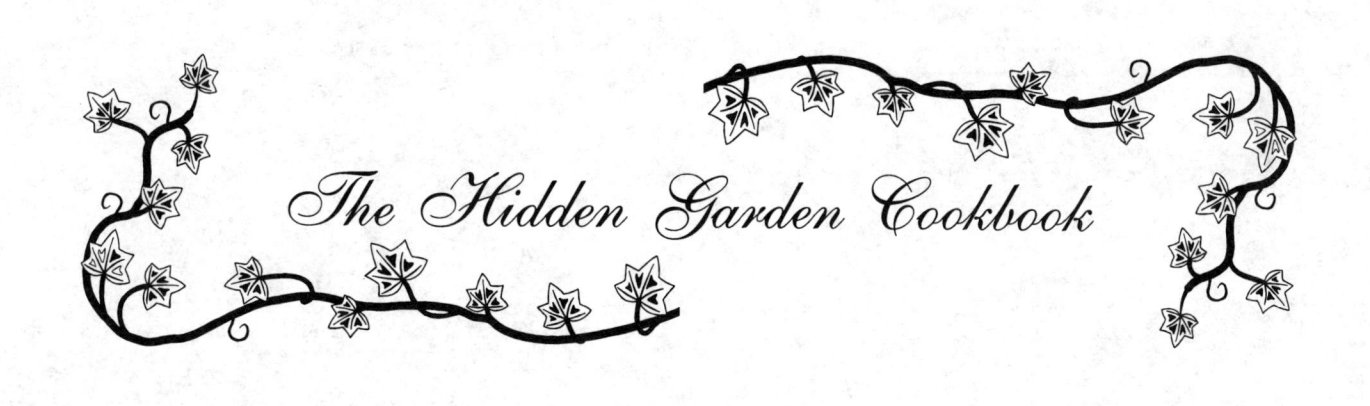

Polenta

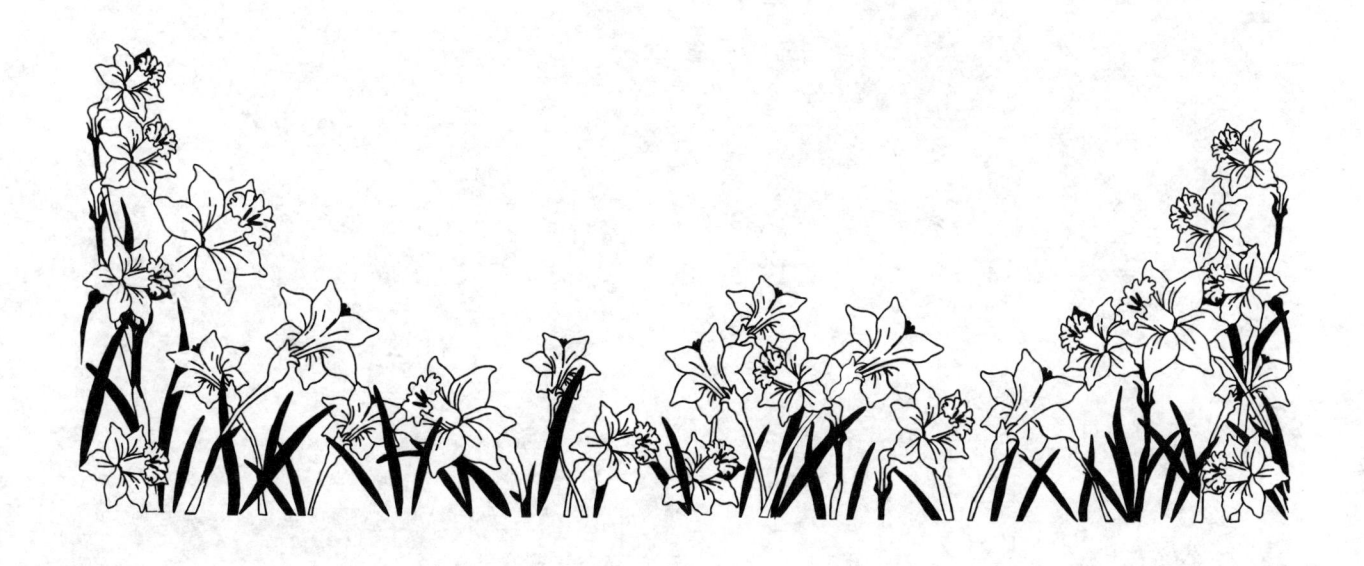

The "Real" Italian Country Style Polenta

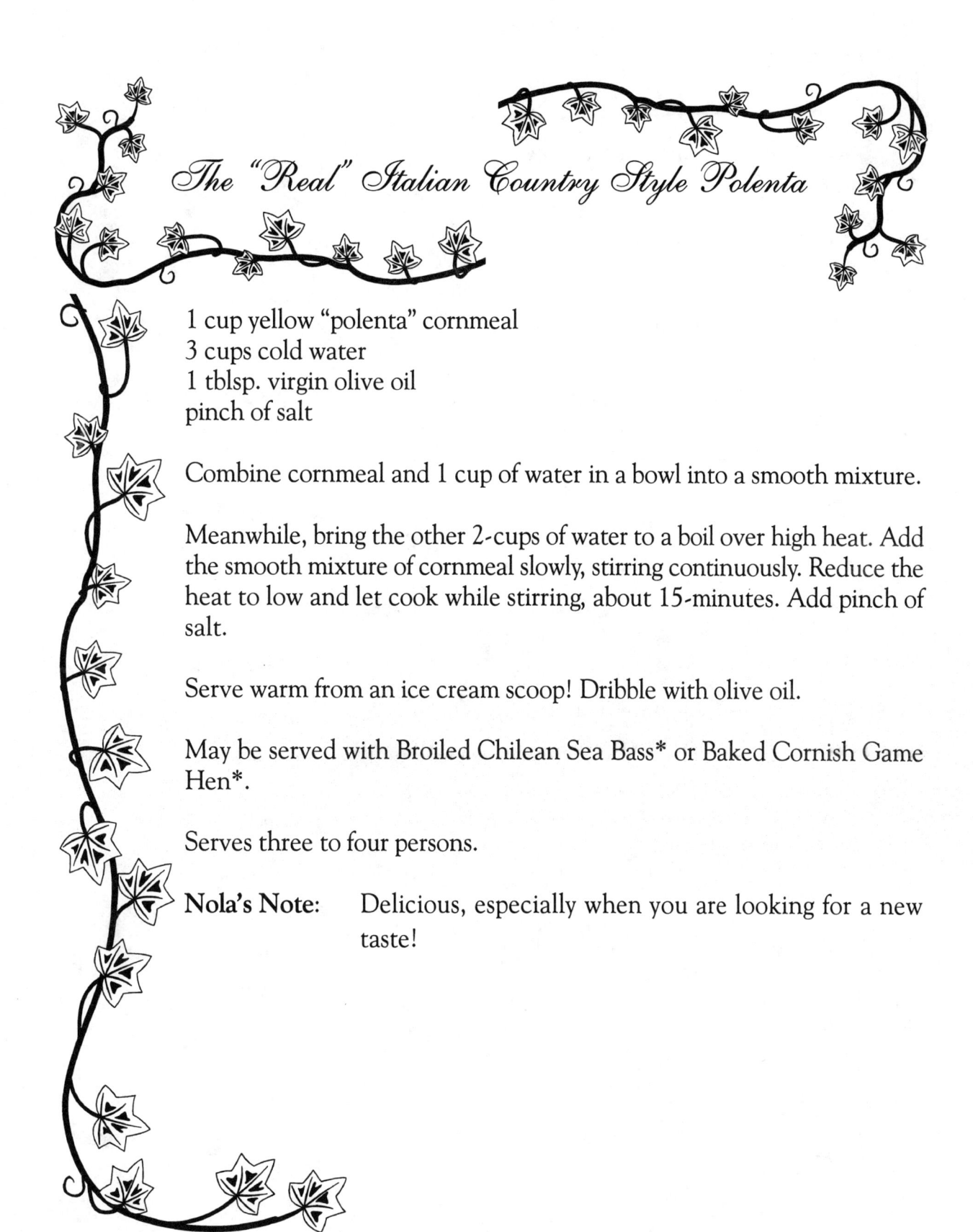

1 cup yellow "polenta" cornmeal
3 cups cold water
1 tblsp. virgin olive oil
pinch of salt

Combine cornmeal and 1 cup of water in a bowl into a smooth mixture.

Meanwhile, bring the other 2-cups of water to a boil over high heat. Add the smooth mixture of cornmeal slowly, stirring continuously. Reduce the heat to low and let cook while stirring, about 15-minutes. Add pinch of salt.

Serve warm from an ice cream scoop! Dribble with olive oil.

May be served with Broiled Chilean Sea Bass* or Baked Cornish Game Hen*.

Serves three to four persons.

Nola's Note: Delicious, especially when you are looking for a new taste!

The Hidden Garden Cookbook

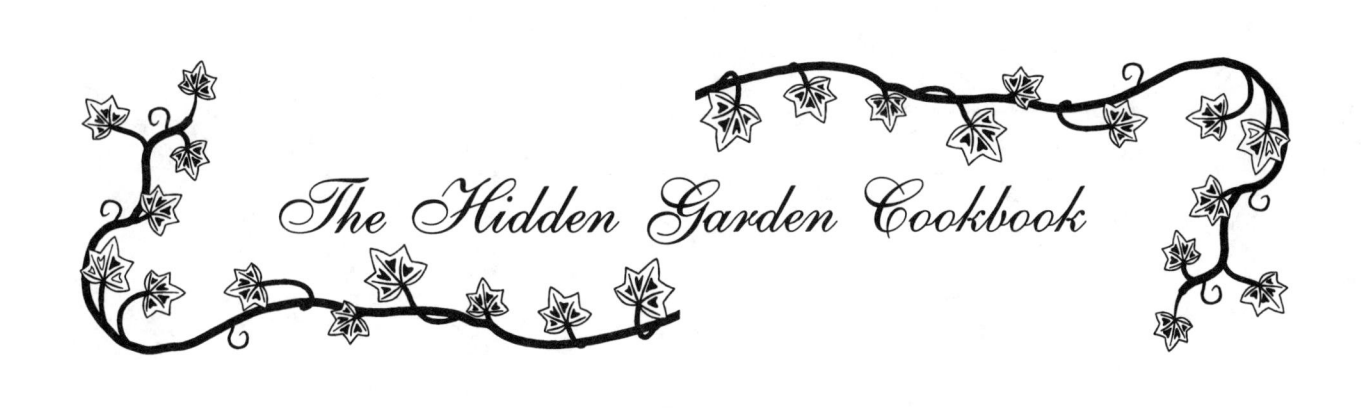

Wild Rice

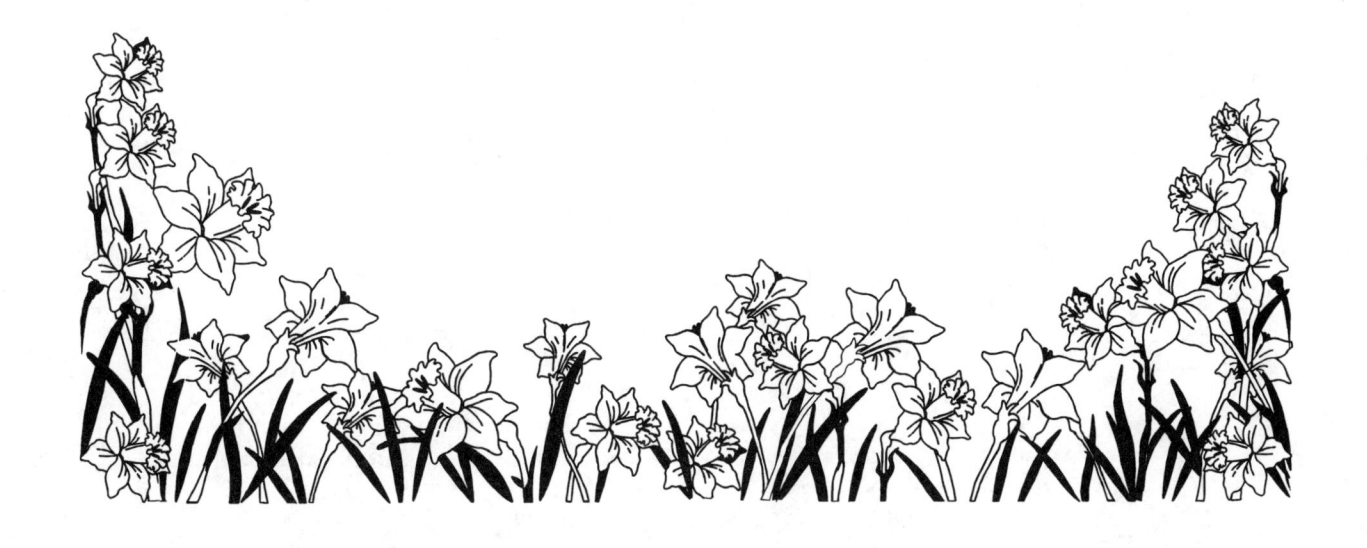

Wild Wild Rice

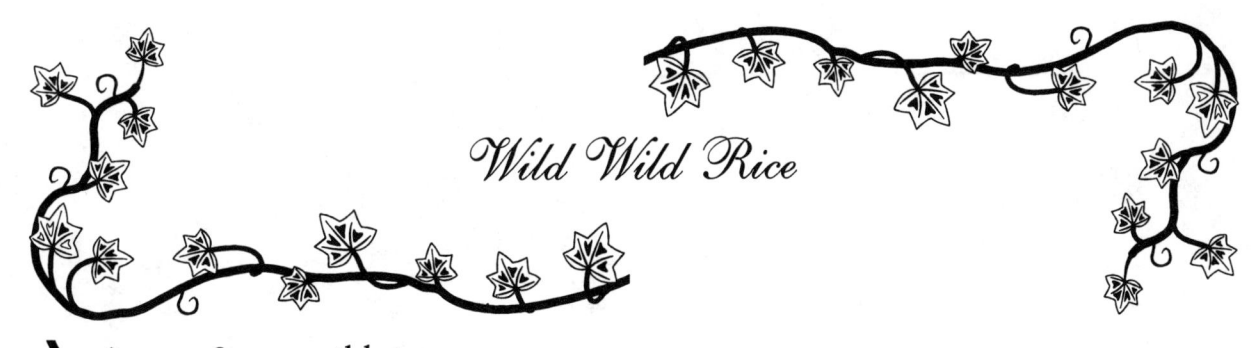

2 cups wild rice
2 tblsp. margarine
1 cup finely-chopped parsley
Pinch of salt & pepper to taste

Wash the wild rice thoroughly. Over high heat, let boil in a heavy pan covered with water. Lower the heat, stir continuously and let simmer, uncovered until grains pop open. Drain and let cool.

Heat margarine in a medium pan, add rice. Sauté well for at 2-3 minutes. Add parsley.

Serve warm. Goes well with Baked Norwegian Salmon* and Grilled Japanese Eggplant*.

Serves five or six.

Nola's Note: You need salt. The wild rice has no flavor otherwise.

The Hidden Garden Cookbook

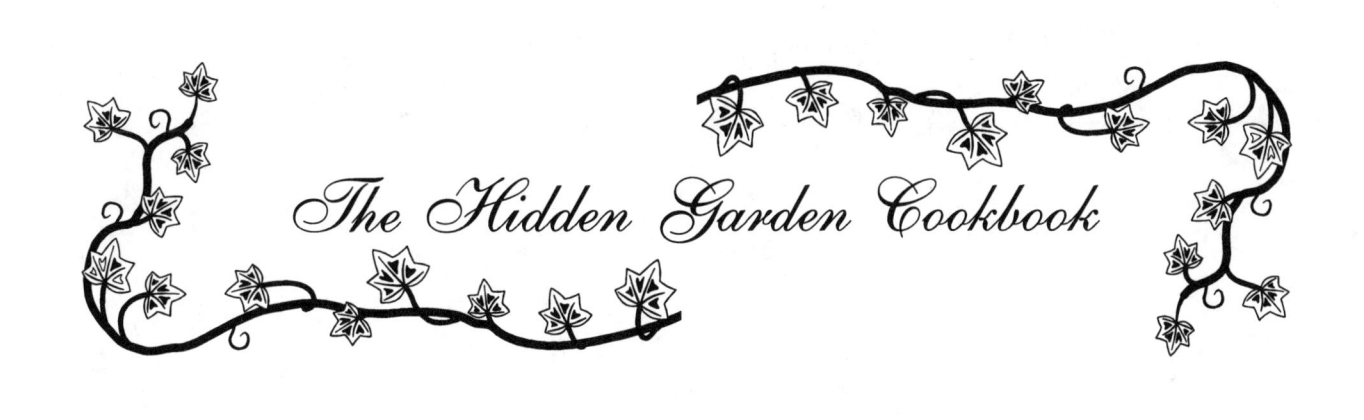

Veggies

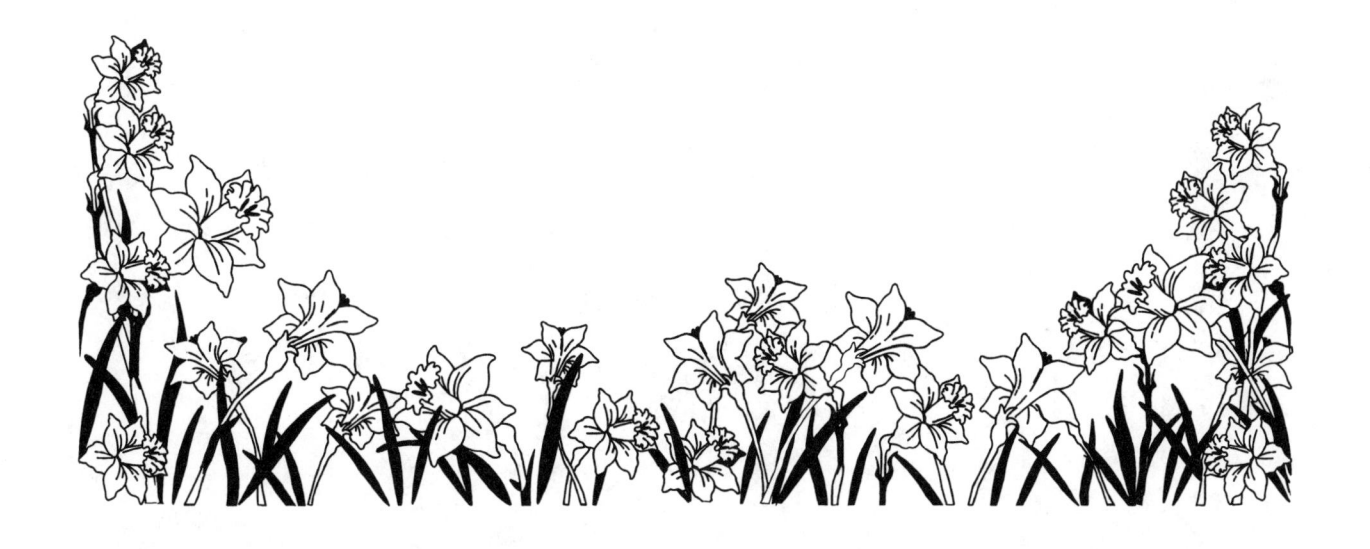

Baked or Grilled Japanese Eggplant

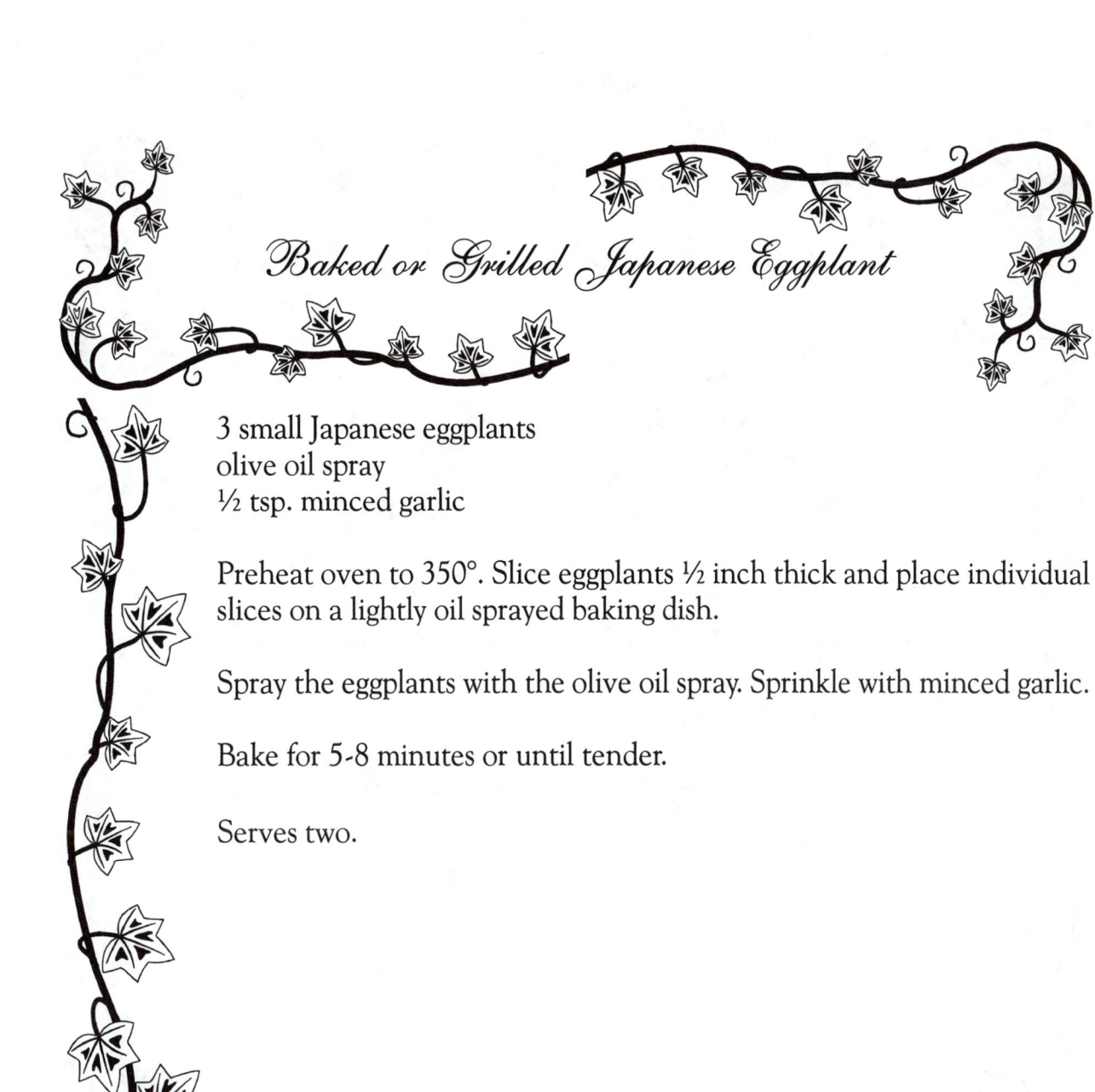

3 small Japanese eggplants
olive oil spray
½ tsp. minced garlic

Preheat oven to 350°. Slice eggplants ½ inch thick and place individual slices on a lightly oil sprayed baking dish.

Spray the eggplants with the olive oil spray. Sprinkle with minced garlic.

Bake for 5-8 minutes or until tender.

Serves two.

Baked Scallopini Squash with Dill Weed

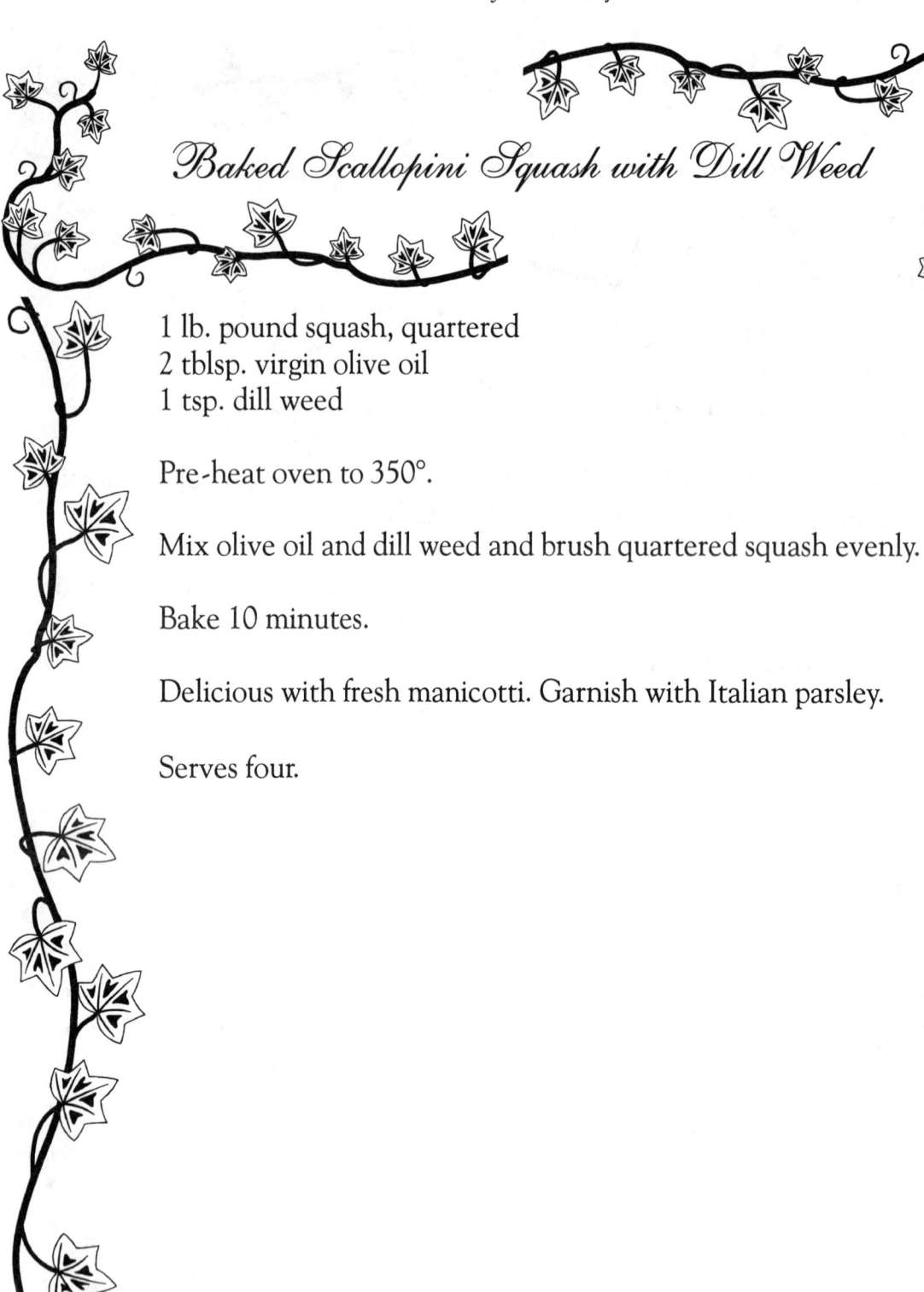

1 lb. pound squash, quartered
2 tblsp. virgin olive oil
1 tsp. dill weed

Pre-heat oven to 350°.

Mix olive oil and dill weed and brush quartered squash evenly.

Bake 10 minutes.

Delicious with fresh manicotti. Garnish with Italian parsley.

Serves four.

Steamed Zucchini with Fresh Basil

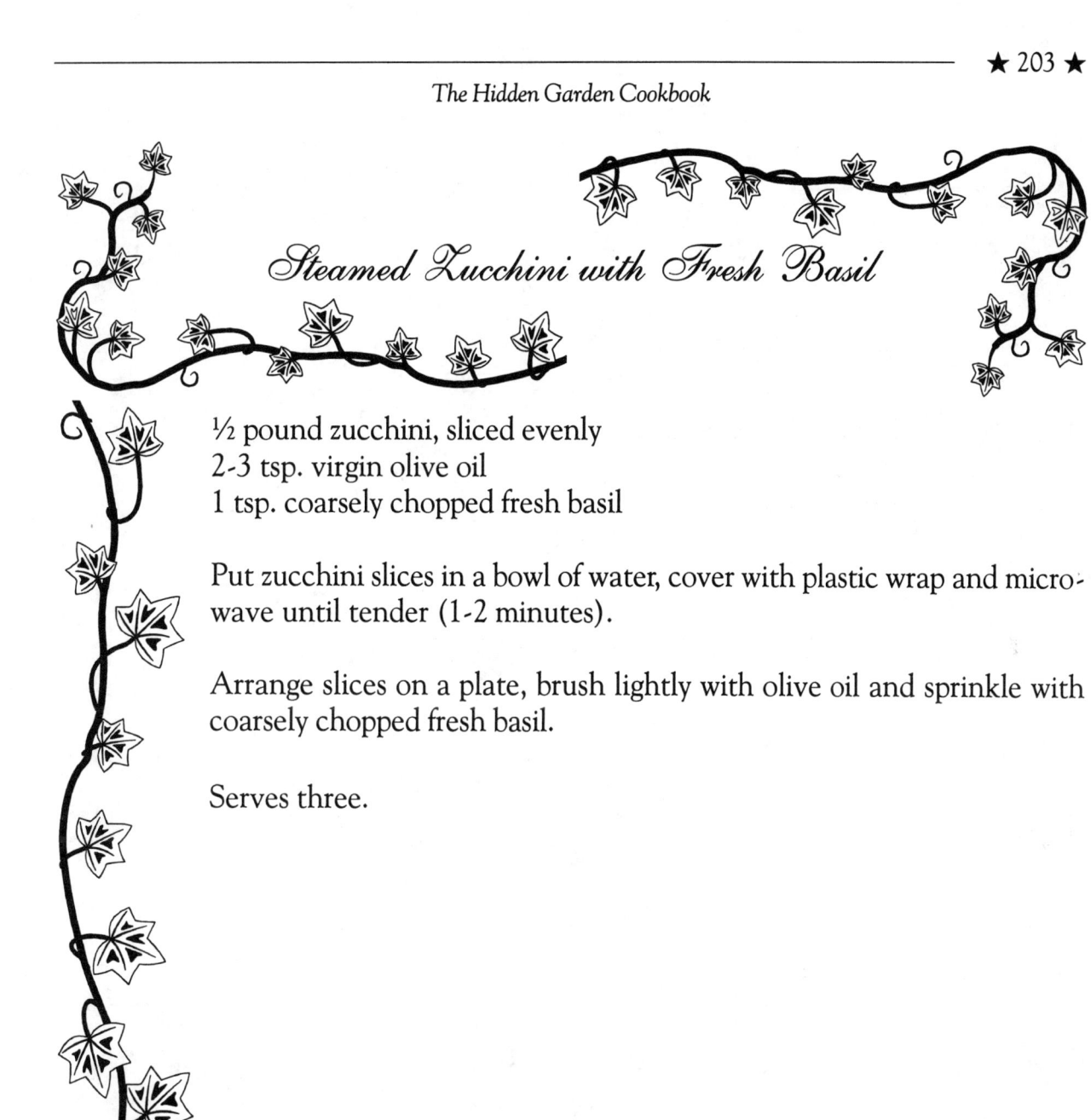

½ pound zucchini, sliced evenly
2-3 tsp. virgin olive oil
1 tsp. coarsely chopped fresh basil

Put zucchini slices in a bowl of water, cover with plastic wrap and microwave until tender (1-2 minutes).

Arrange slices on a plate, brush lightly with olive oil and sprinkle with coarsely chopped fresh basil.

Serves three.

The Hidden Garden Cookbook

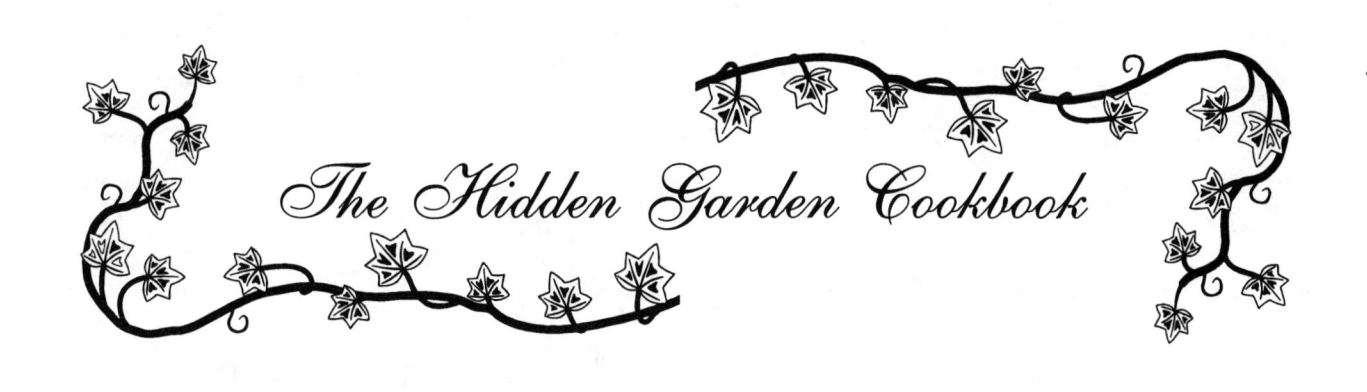

Tea Bread
&
Muffins

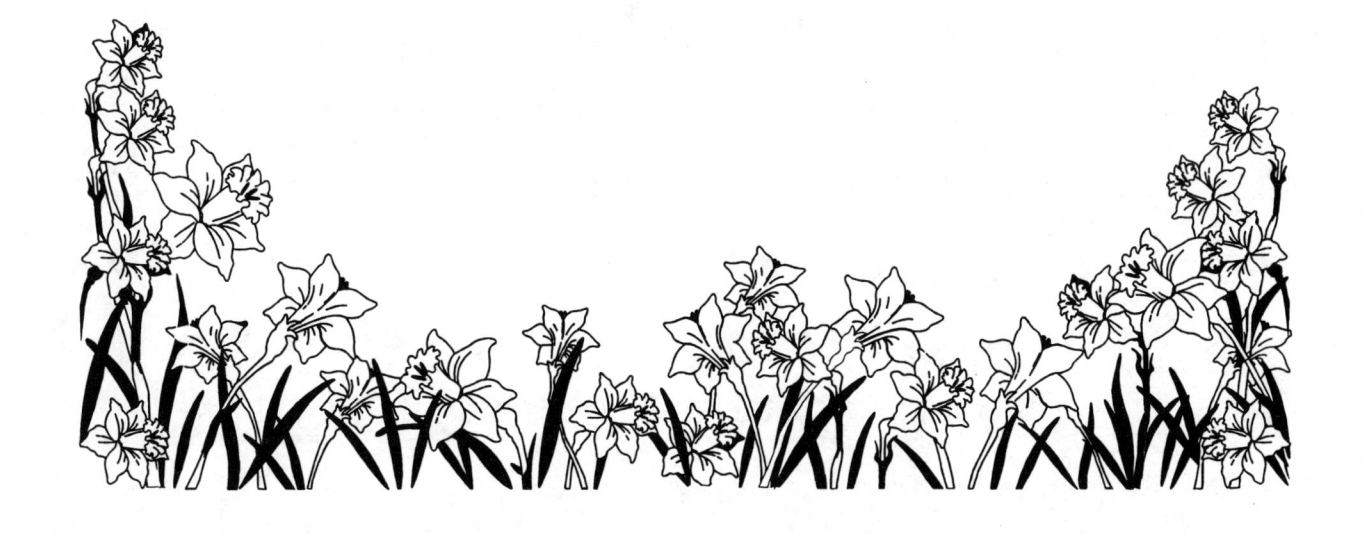

Banana-Fruit Tea Bread

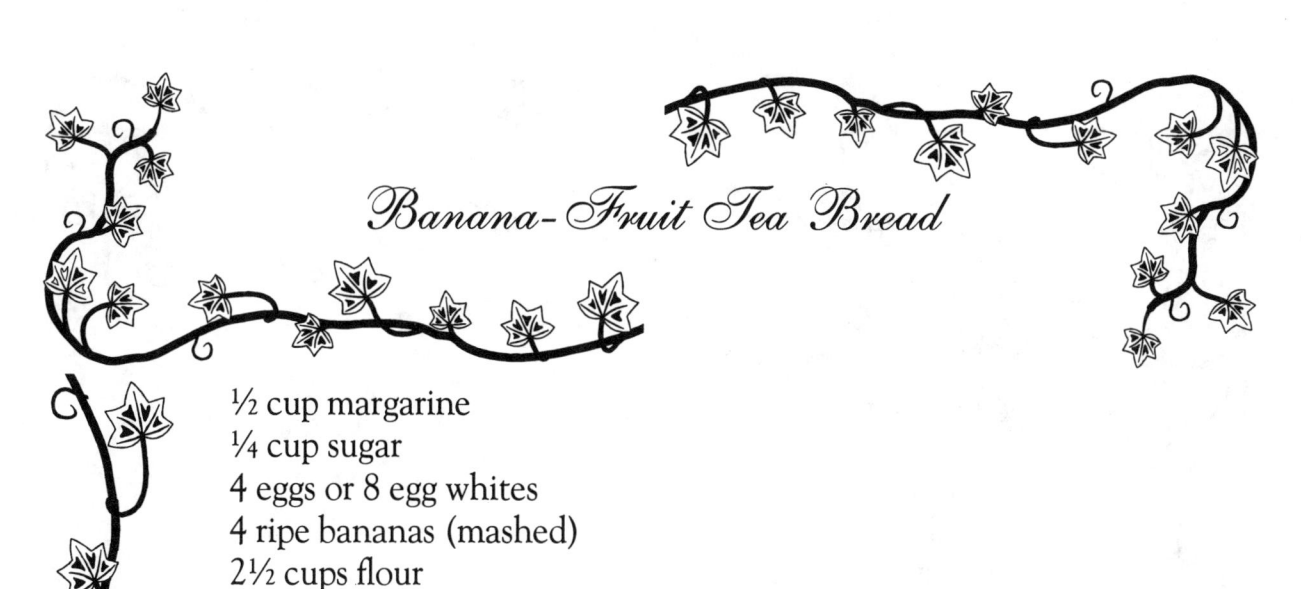

½ cup margarine
¼ cup sugar
4 eggs or 8 egg whites
4 ripe bananas (mashed)
2½ cups flour
2 tsp baking soda
½ cup dried pitted cherries**
½ cup golden raisins**
½ cup currants**
½ cup chopped walnuts (omit for face surgery patients)

Preheat oven to 325°. Grease and flour loaf pans or bundt.
Cream margarine and sugar until fluffy. Add well-beaten egg whites and mashed bananas. Add flour and baking soda. *Do not over-mix.* Strain soaked cherries, golden raisins and currants.
Gently fold fruits into bread mixture. Bake for 35-40 minutes or until a wooden pick inserted in center comes out clean.

Serve sliced and lightly toasted.
Serves six to ten.
**Soak in water for 10 minutes.

Nola's Note: Our desserts and breads use only the minimum amount of sugar. If necessary you may want to add more sugar, but you will lose the natural fruit flavors when adding sugar. So go carefully.

Grandmother's Oat Bran Muffins

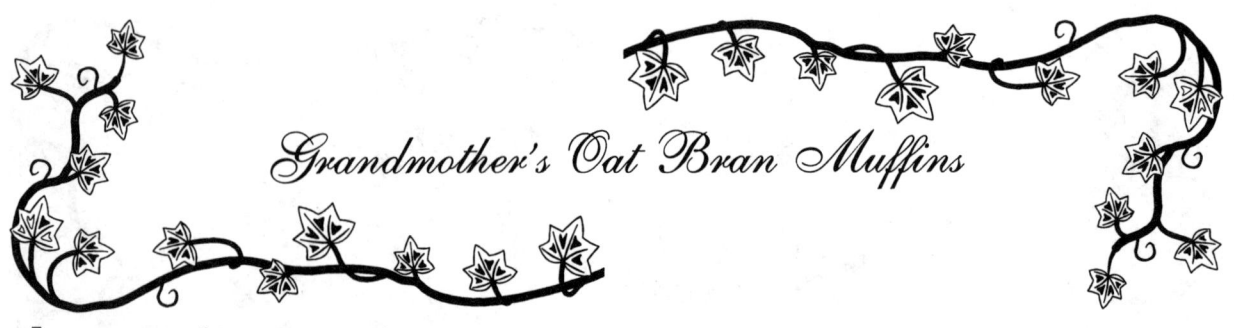

1 cup margarine
1 cup sugar
10 egg whites
2 cups light sour cream
3 cups flour
1 cup oat bran flakes
3 tsp. baking soda
1 cup Kellog's All Bran
2 cups buttermilk
2 tsp baking powder
2 cups currants
1½ cups chopped walnuts

Preheat oven to 400°. Cream margarine and sugar, set aside. Beat egg whites and sour cream at high speed for 3 minutes. In a large bowl, mix flour, oat bran flakes, baking soda, Kellog's All Bran, baking powder and buttermilk. Mix well. Add to beaten egg white-sour cream mixture. Beat at medium speed while adding creamed margarine-sugar mixture. Blend well.

Add currants and chopped walnuts. Stir well, using rubber spatula.

Pour batter into greased mini-muffin pan and bake for 20 minutes or until an inserted wooden pick comes out clean. Let cool for 5 minutes then transfer onto a cooling rack to cool completely.

Heat in toaster oven before serving.

Makes 48 mini-muffins.

The Hidden Garden Cookbook

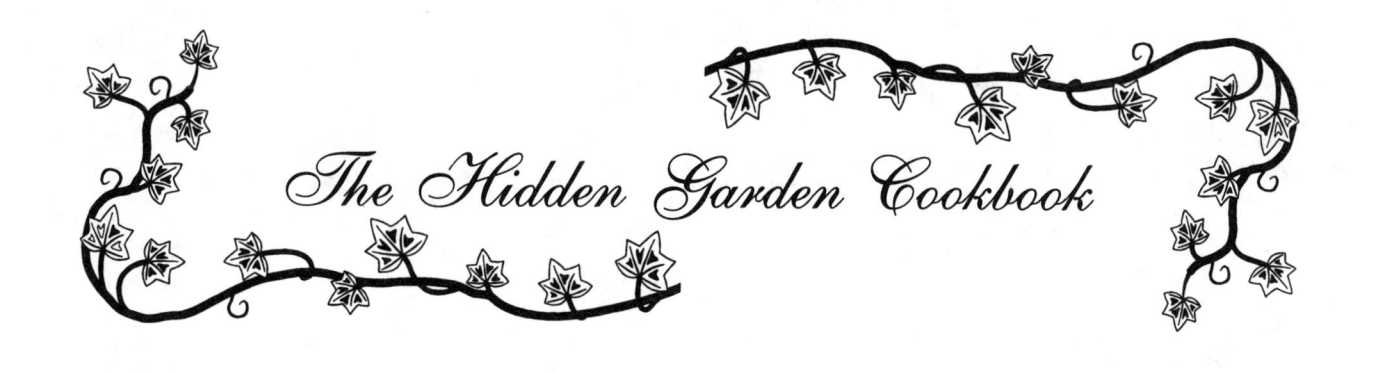

Cakes & Pies

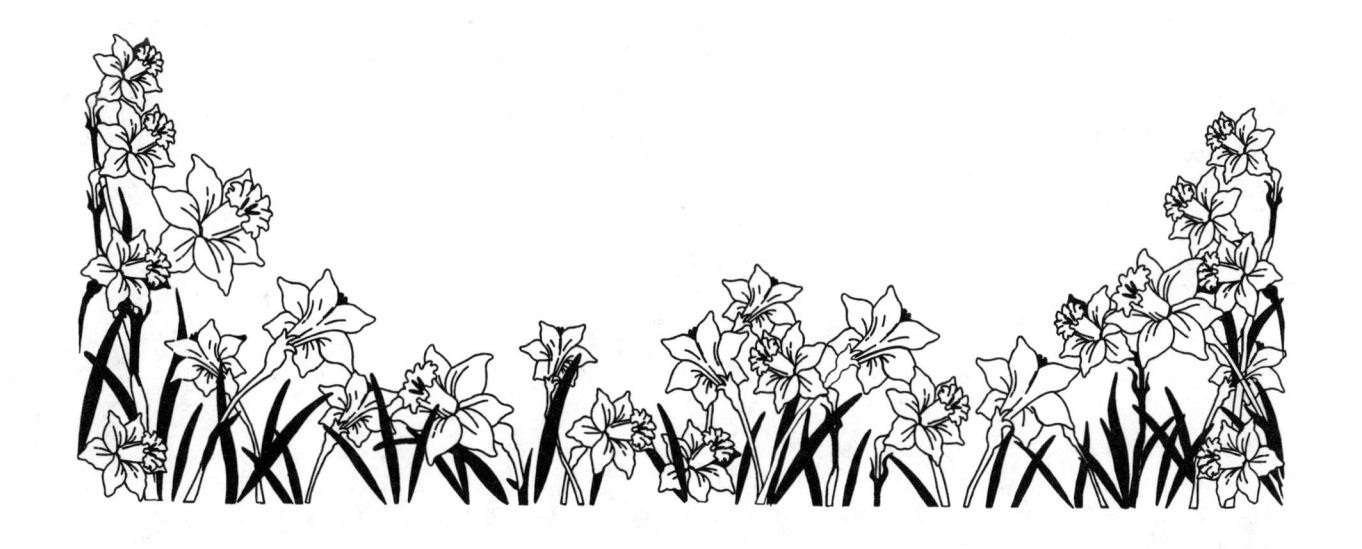

Zangy Lemon Poppy Seed Cake

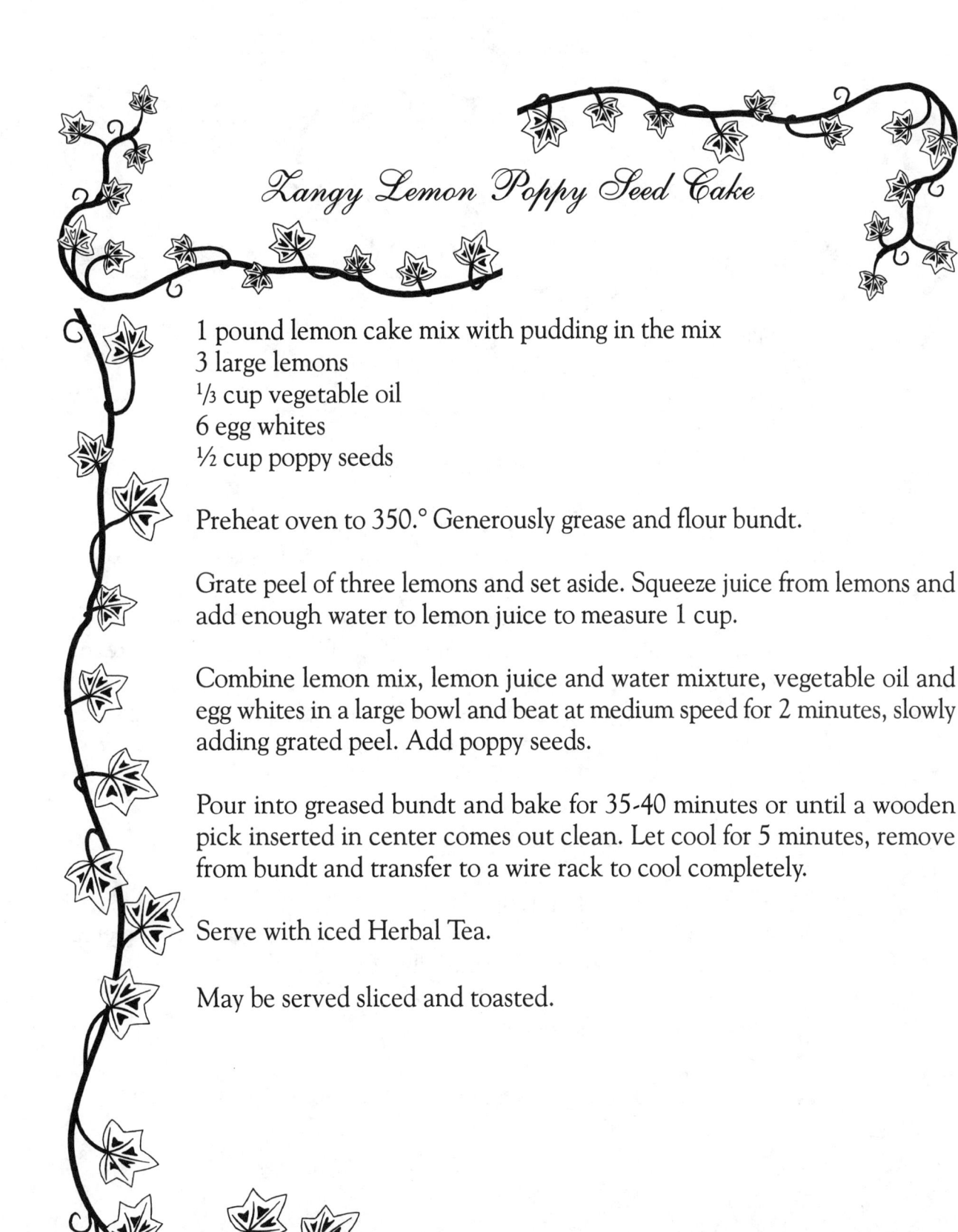

1 pound lemon cake mix with pudding in the mix
3 large lemons
1/3 cup vegetable oil
6 egg whites
1/2 cup poppy seeds

Preheat oven to 350.° Generously grease and flour bundt.

Grate peel of three lemons and set aside. Squeeze juice from lemons and add enough water to lemon juice to measure 1 cup.

Combine lemon mix, lemon juice and water mixture, vegetable oil and egg whites in a large bowl and beat at medium speed for 2 minutes, slowly adding grated peel. Add poppy seeds.

Pour into greased bundt and bake for 35-40 minutes or until a wooden pick inserted in center comes out clean. Let cool for 5 minutes, remove from bundt and transfer to a wire rack to cool completely.

Serve with iced Herbal Tea.

May be served sliced and toasted.

Nola's 4th of July Apple Pie

Pie Pastry*
6-8 large tart apples, peeled, cored and thinly sliced
1-2 tblsp. sugar
1 tblsp. lemon juice
½ tsp. vanilla powder or ½ tsp. ground cinnamon

Preheat oven to 425°. Roll out pastry for bottom crust and line a 9-inch pie pan. Cover with foil and bake for 10 minutes. Remove foil. Cool.

In a large bowl, combine sugar, vanilla powder or cinnamon. Add the sliced apples. Sprinkle with lemon juice. Toss. Pile the apple mixture into the cooled bottom pastry crust. With your hands, gently press the apple mixture down into the pie pan. Pile additional apple mixture into pan and press down again. Apples should be very high, mountain-like, in the pie pan.

Cover with pastry strips, trim and flute the edges.

Bake for 20 minutes, then reduce heat to 350° and continue to bake for 30-40 minutes more. Do not overbake. Apples are tender when pierced with a knife. If crust browns too rapidly, cover crust with foil.

Sprinkle with powdered sugar.

Nola's Note: Taste apples first for tartness before adding sugar.

Nola's Incredible Blueberry Pie

Pie Pastry*
4 qts. fresh ripe blueberries
2 tblsp. granulated tapioca or flour
1 tblsp. sugar (optional)

Preheat oven to 424°. Roll out pastry for bottom crust and line a 10-inch pie pan. Cover with foil and bake for 10 minutes. Let cool.

In a very large bowl, gently toss the tapioca, sugar and berries. Pile the berries into the cooled bottom pastry crust. Gently press the berries down into the pie pan *with your hands,* with each addition of berries, gently press again to compact the berries together.

Cover with top crust, trim and flute the edges. Cut 3-4 vents.

Bake for 25 minutes, then reduce heat to 350°, and continue to bake for another 35 minutes.

Nola's Note: Taste berries first for tartness before adding   sugar.

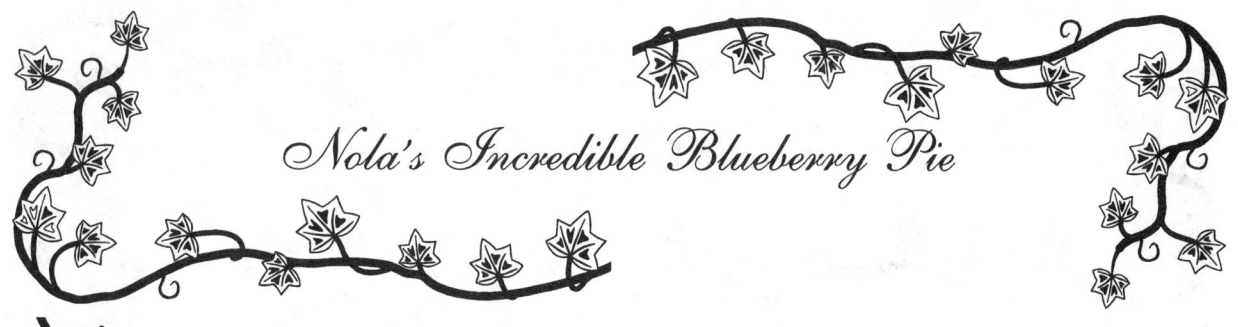

Pear Tart

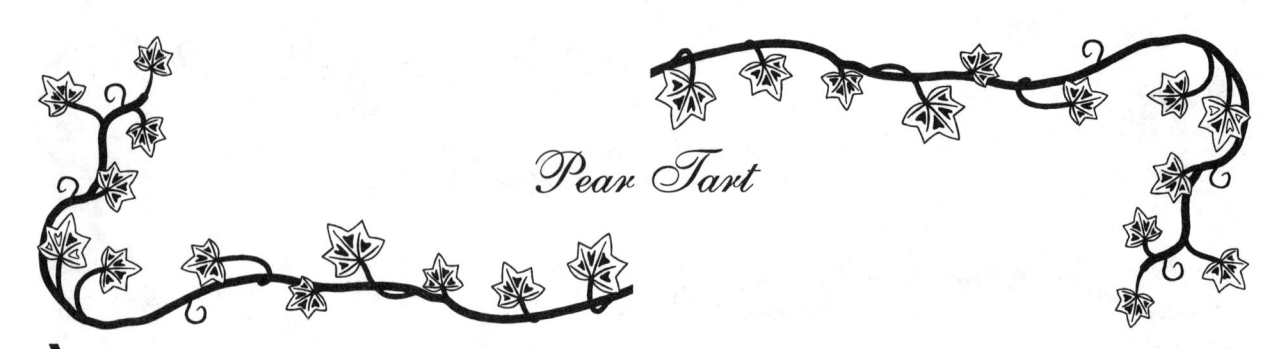

Pie Pastry*
6-8 Bartlett pears, peeled, cored and thinly sliced
1-2 tblsp. sugar
1 tblsp. lemon juice
1 tblsp. vanilla extract
¼ cup chopped pistachio nuts
½ cup apricot glaze

Prepare bottom Pie Pastry* (no top crust is used)

Line prepared bottom Pie Pastry with "fanned" slices of pear. Sprinkle with lemon juice and sugar. Sprinkle vanilla extract lightly. Continue with additional layers until all pear slices are used. Top layer should resemble a pretty "fan" of sliced pears. Cover crust trim with foil.

Bake at 350° for 40-45 minutes. Do not overbake. Remove crust foil last 10-15 minutes.

Cool. Sprinkle apricot glaze and chopped pistachio nuts.

Glaze: Scoop ¼ cup apricot jam into saucepan. Add ¼ cup water. Boil. Pour glaze over pear tart.

Nola's Note: Pears are wonderful. Once you cook with fresh pears, you will never STOP!!

Pie Pastry

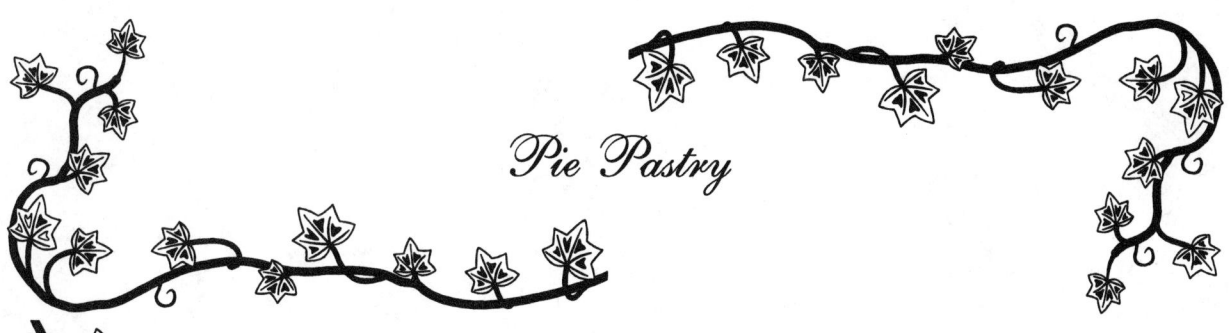

1¼ cups flour
1 tblsp. sugar
¼ tsp. salt
½ cup Crisco
2 tblsp. or more ice cold water

Place into food processor the flour, sugar and salt. Cut the Crisco into 4 or 5 pieces and add into the processor. Mix for 15 seconds. Add water while mixing again for 15 seconds. When the dough sticks together when "pinched," it is ready. If too dry, add more water. Form dough into a ball and then flatten the ball into a fat pancake.

Roll dough out onto a floured linen kitchen towel. Transfer the rolled-out dough to the pie pan. Trim edges. Save extra dough for strips to be used as a lattice top (if needed).

Preheat oven to 425°. Cover bottom crust with foil and back for 10 minutes. Remove foil. Cool.

Fill pie pan with selected filling. Cover top with lattice stips (if needed).

Bake according to recipe.

The Hidden Garden Cookbook

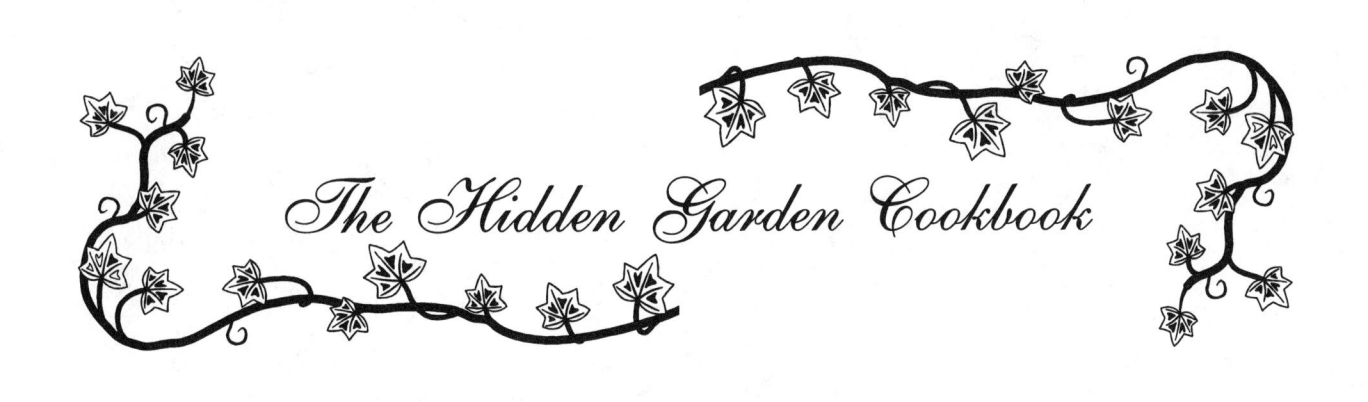

Shakes

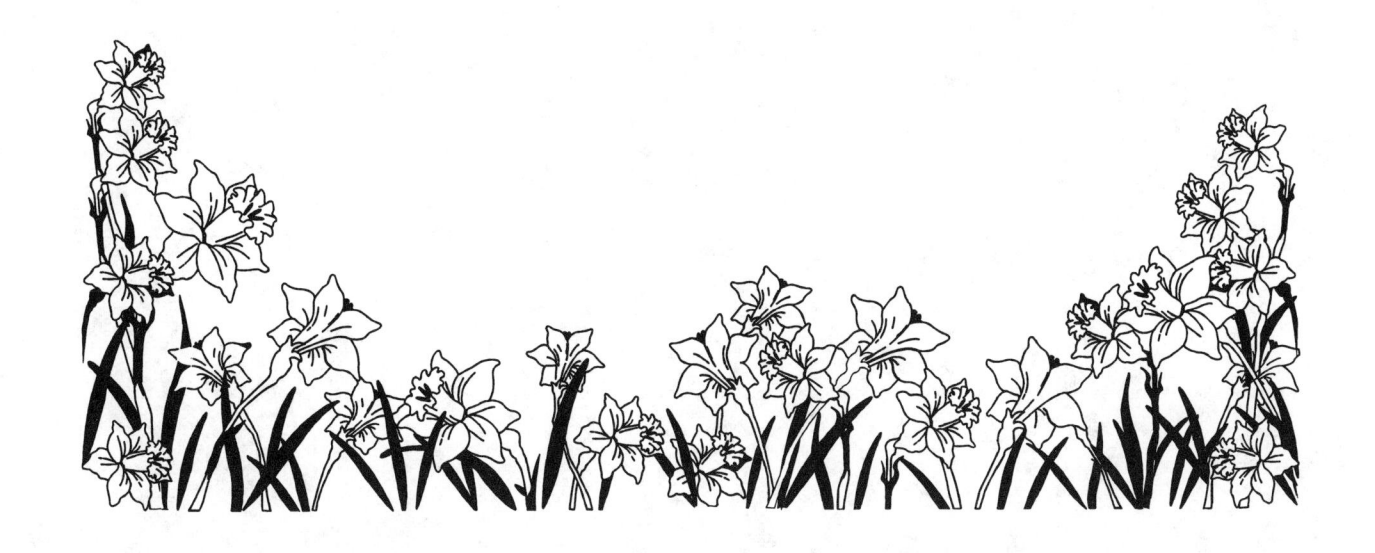

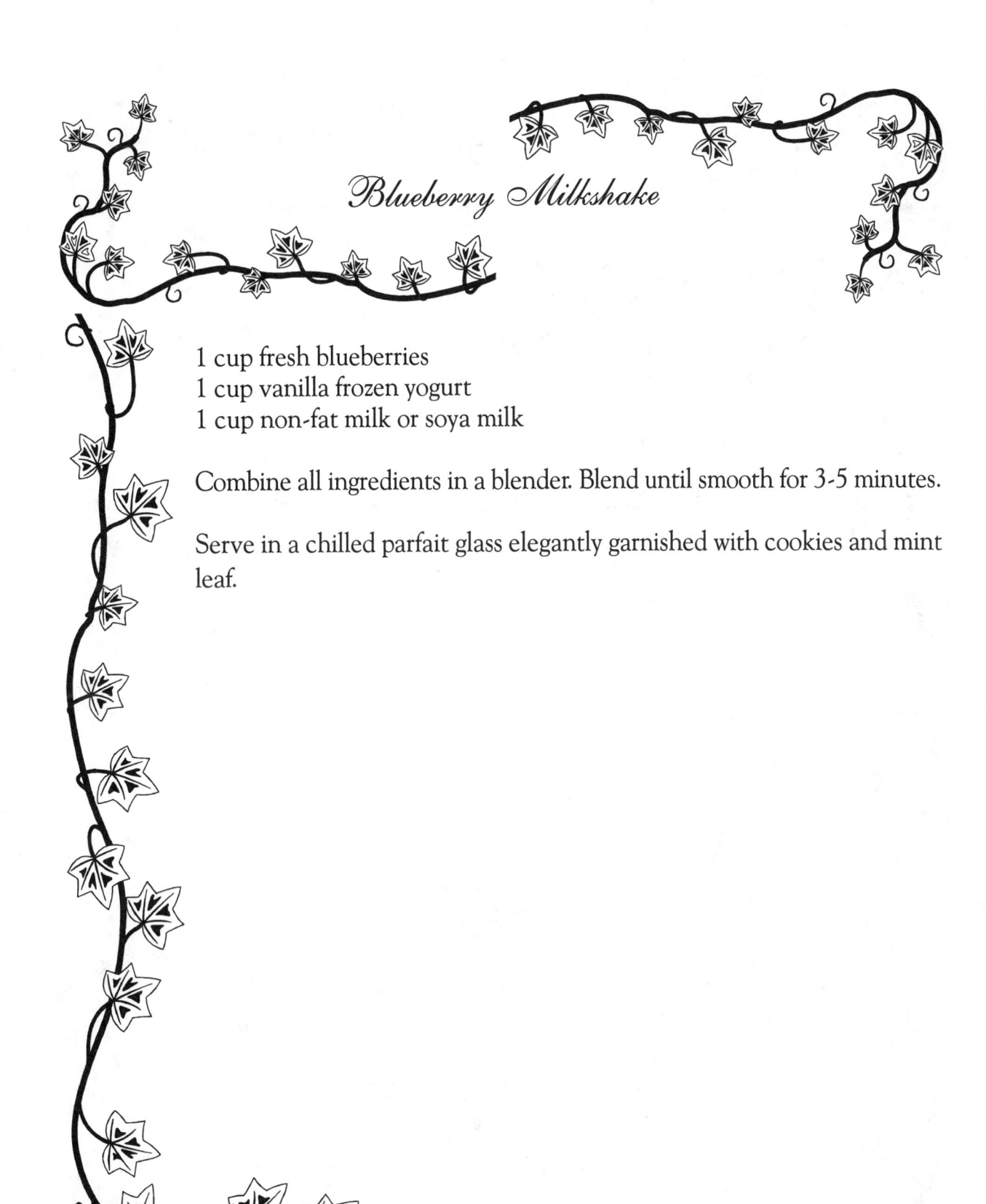

Blueberry Milkshake

1 cup fresh blueberries
1 cup vanilla frozen yogurt
1 cup non-fat milk or soya milk

Combine all ingredients in a blender. Blend until smooth for 3-5 minutes.

Serve in a chilled parfait glass elegantly garnished with cookies and mint leaf.

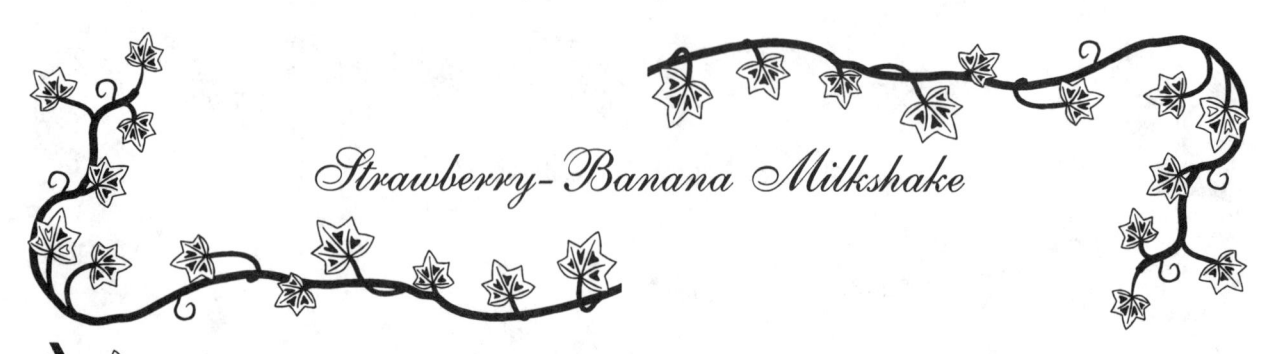

Strawberry-Banana Milkshake

1 cup freshly-cut or sliced strawberries
½ banana, sliced
1 cup vanilla frozen yogurt
1 cup non-fat milk or soya milk

Combine all ingredients in a blender. Blend until smooth for 3-5 minutes.

Garnish with whole fresh strawberries and sprig of mint. Serve in a tall glass.

Dr. Fisher's Shake

1 cup sliced fresh strawberries
½ or whole banana
1 cup vanilla ice cream
1 or 2 eggs
1 cup milk

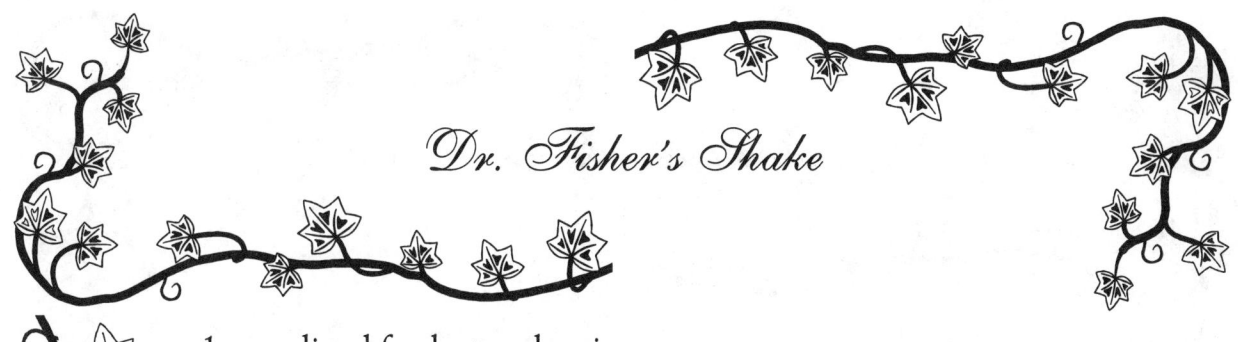

Combine all ingredients in a blender. Blend until smooth for 3-5 minutes.

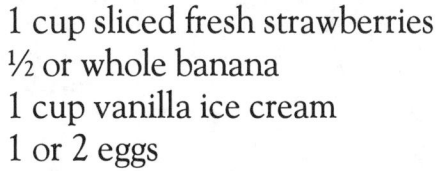

Garnish with mint leaf and fresh whole strawberry.

Serve in a chilled parfait glass.

Nola's Note: This is a "killer" milkshake! Male guests at The Hidden Garden love this for Tea Time and Midnight Snack

Chocolate Milkshake

1 cup vanilla frozen yogurt
1 cup chocolate frozen yogurt
½ cup non-fat milk or soya milk
1 tblsp. Hershey's Syrup (optional)

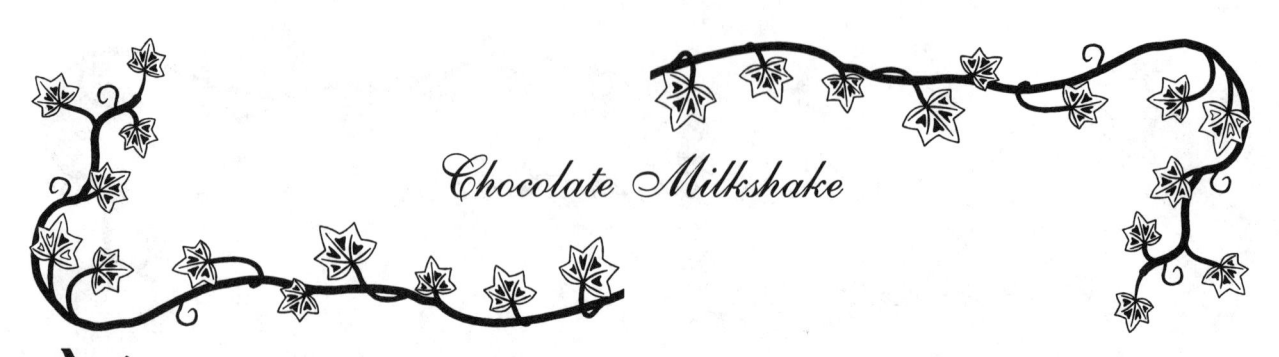

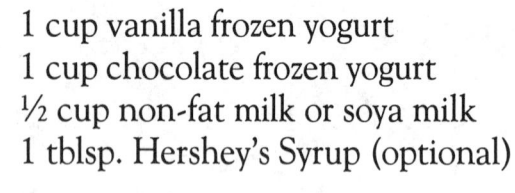

Combine all ingredients in a blender. Blend until smooth for 3-5 minutes.

Serve in a chilled parfait glass, elegantly garnished with cookies and mint leaf.

Diane's Fruit Smoothie

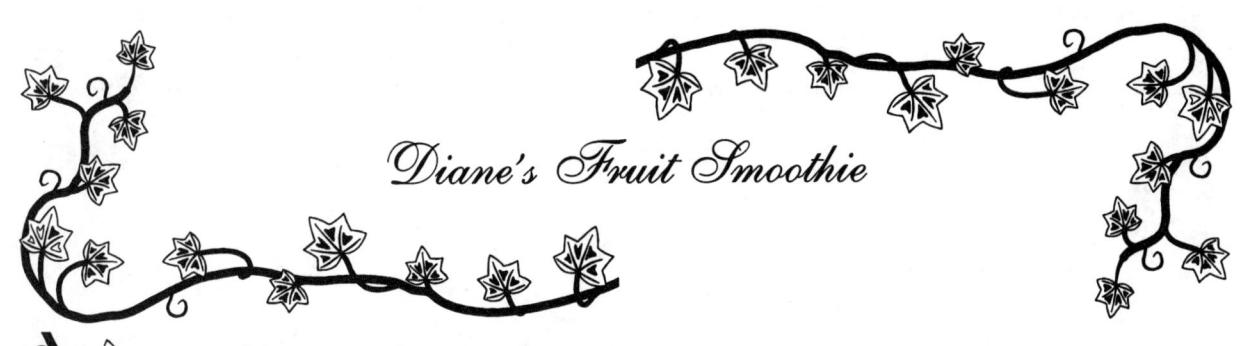

3 tblsp. strawberry sorbet
½ cup apple juice
½ cup chopped fruits (banana, cantaloupe, pear, peaches, etc.)

Mix all ingredients in a blender and puree until smooth.

Delicious and appetizing.

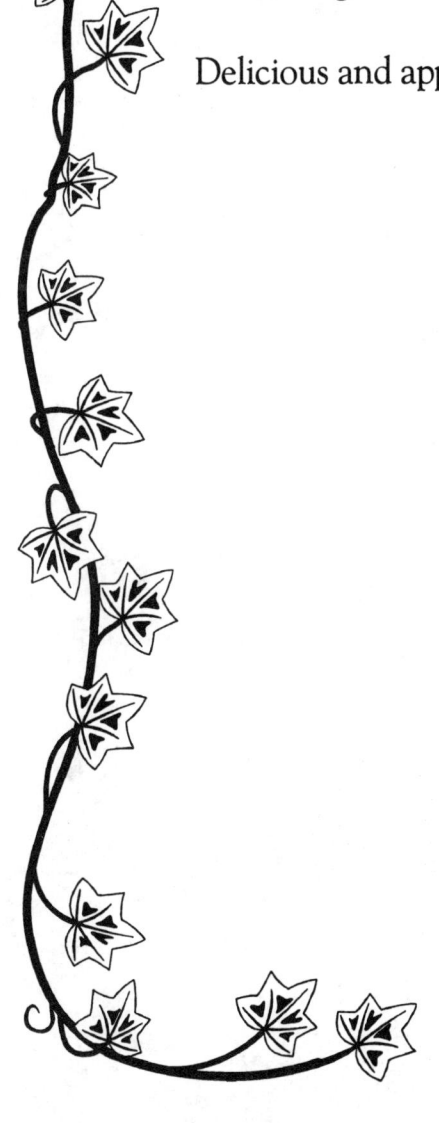

The Hidden Garden Cookbook

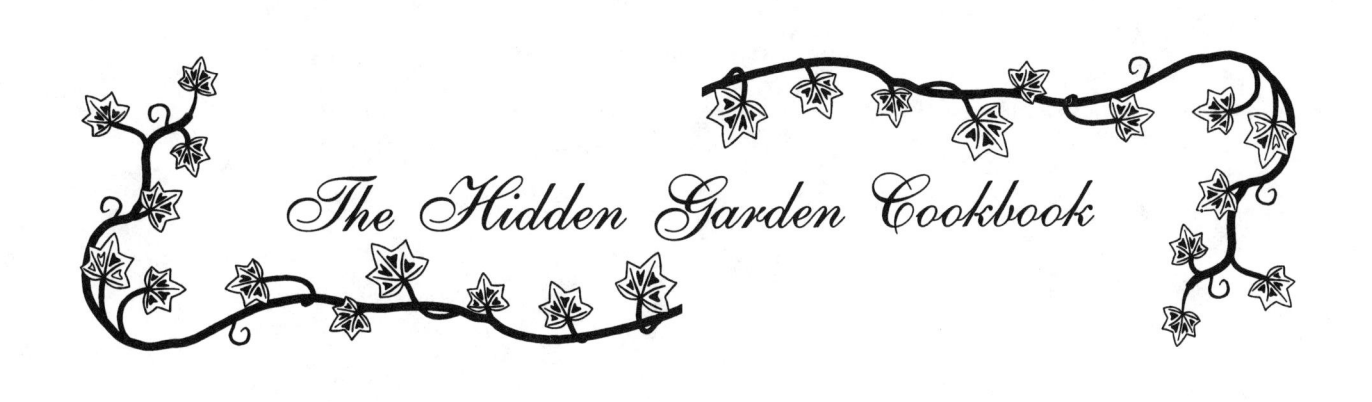

Chocolates

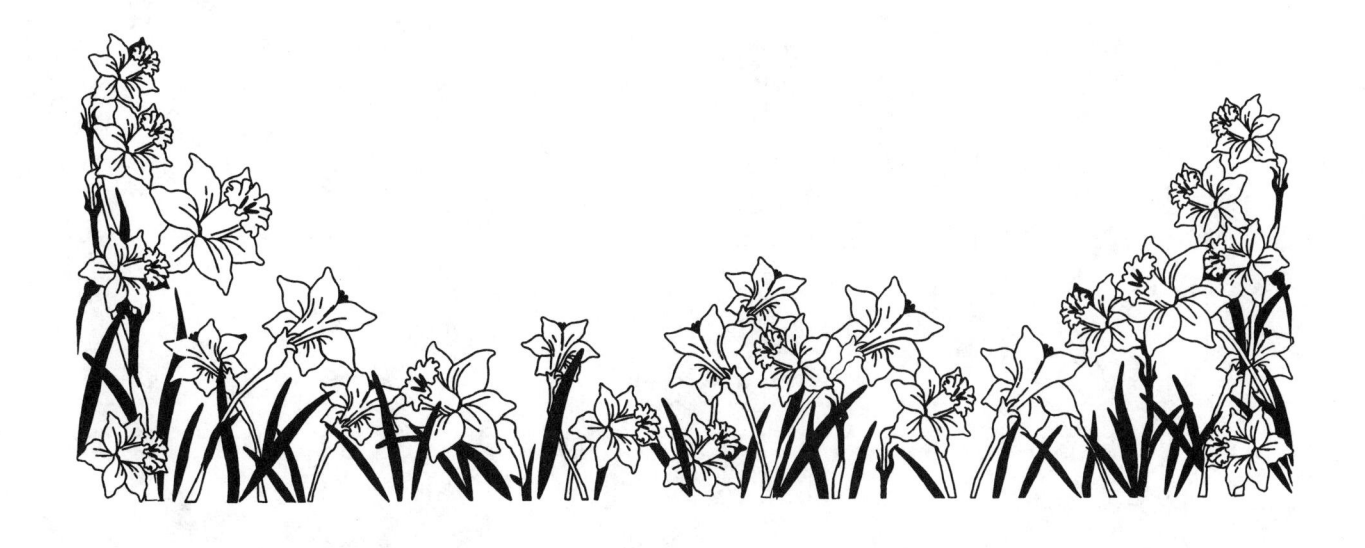

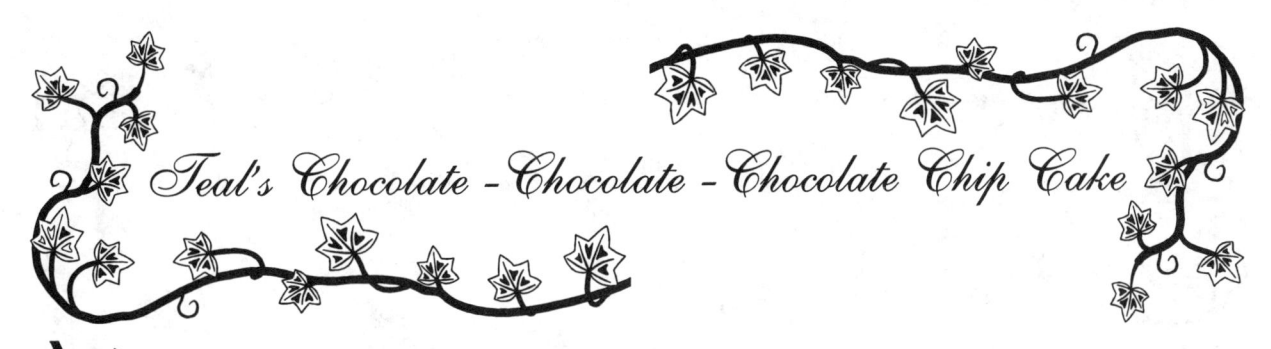

Teal's Chocolate-Chocolate-Chocolate Chip Cake

1 pound chocolate cake mix w/pudding in the mix
1 1/3 cups water
1/3 cup vegetable oil
6 egg whites
6 oz. semi-sweet chocolate chip "morsels"

Preheat oven to 350°. Generously grease and flour bundt pan.

Combine cake mix, water, vegetable oil and egg whites in a large bowl and beat on medium speed for 2-minutes.

Spread evenly 3 oz. chocolate chips in a greased and floured bundt before pouring cake mixture. Add the remaining 3 oz. chocolate chips on top of cake mixture/batter. Let these last chips just gently sink into mixture.

Bake for 35-40 minutes. *Let cool for 10-minutes*, remove from bundt and *transfer to a wire rack* to cool.

Serve warm topped with vanilla ice cream or whipped Custard Sauce* with raspberries garnished around the cake or a sprig of mint.

Serves only eight! Everyone will have seconds!

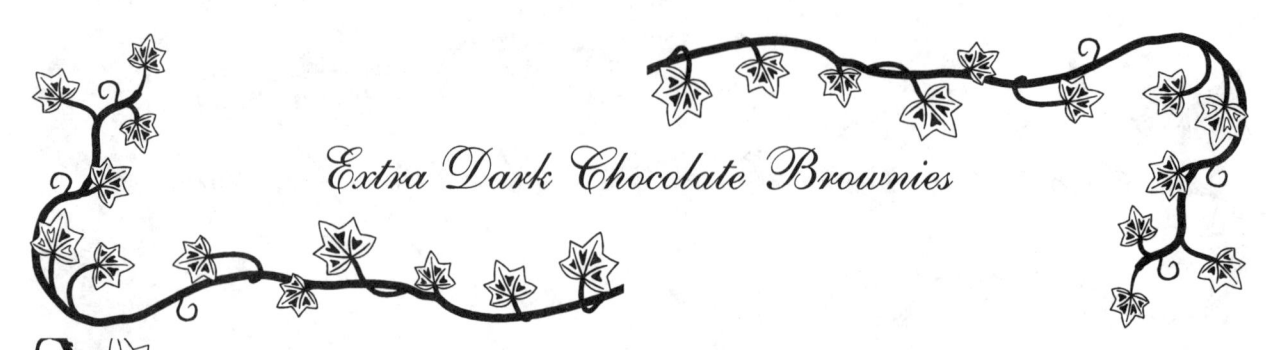

Extra Dark Chocolate Brownies

24 oz. semi-sweet chocolate
3 sticks margarine
6 eggs or 12 egg whites
½ cup sugar
¾ cup all-purpose flour
2 cups walnuts, coarsely chopped
3 tsp. vanilla

Preheat oven to 375°. Line pan with wax paper to make sure brownies won't stick or fall apart when you transfer onto a cooling rack.
Melt semi-sweet chocolate and the margarine in the microwave for 1-minute. Stir and put it back into the microwave for another minute or until melted. Stir with rubber spatula.
Meanwhile, beat eggs or egg whites at high speed gradually adding sugar until it reaches the consistency of soft-peaked whipped cream. Reduce to medium speed, add chocolate mixture and vanilla until well blended. At low speed, add flour just until flour is absorbed. Add coarsely chopped walnuts. Blend with chocolate-flour mixture. Spoon batter evenly into greased 10" baking pan.
Bake for at least 30-40 minutes or until a toothpick inserted comes out clean.
Let cool for an hour before transferring onto a cutting board and cutting into squares.
Serve warm with vanilla ice cream on top.
Makes 20-24 squares.

Nola's Note: Omit walnuts if a facelift patient wants to enjoy these!

Heavenly Chocolate Mousse with Creme Fraiche

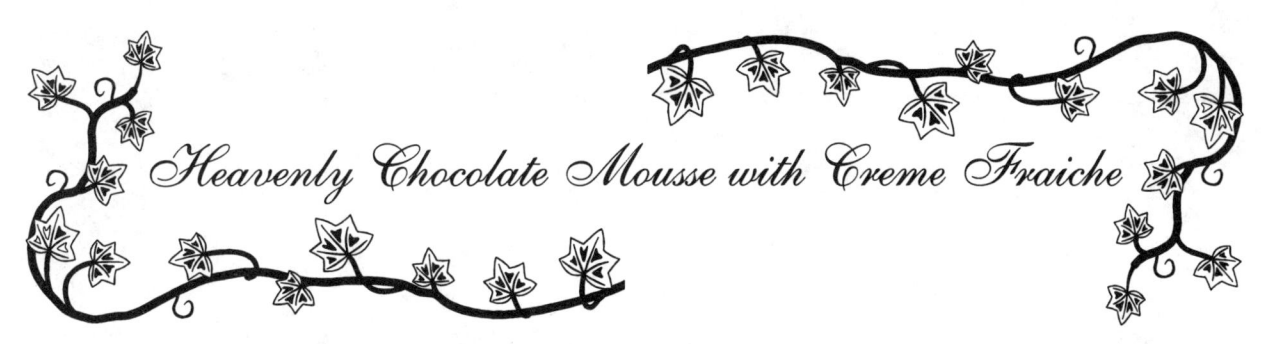

1 pound semi-sweet baking chocolate squares
1½ cups heavy whipping cream
¼ cup strong coffee
½ cup margarine
8 large egg whites

In a small bowl, beat heavy cream at high speed until stiff peaks form. Refrigerate for 30-45 minutes.

Melt chocolate squares and margarine for 1 minute. Add strong coffee, stir and put in microwave for another 1 minute or until chocolate is melted. Mix gently, using a rubber spatula.

Beat egg whites at high speed until soft peaks form. Fold stiff whites into chocolate mixture. Then fold whipped cream into chocolate-egg whites mixture until blended.

Transfer into a dessert bowl or individual dessert cups and refrigerate for 3-4 hours.

Serve with slices of fresh strawberries, topped with Creme Fraiche* and garnished with mint leaves.

Nola's Note: This is a recipe in which the heavy whipping cream must be used.

The Hidden Garden Cookbook

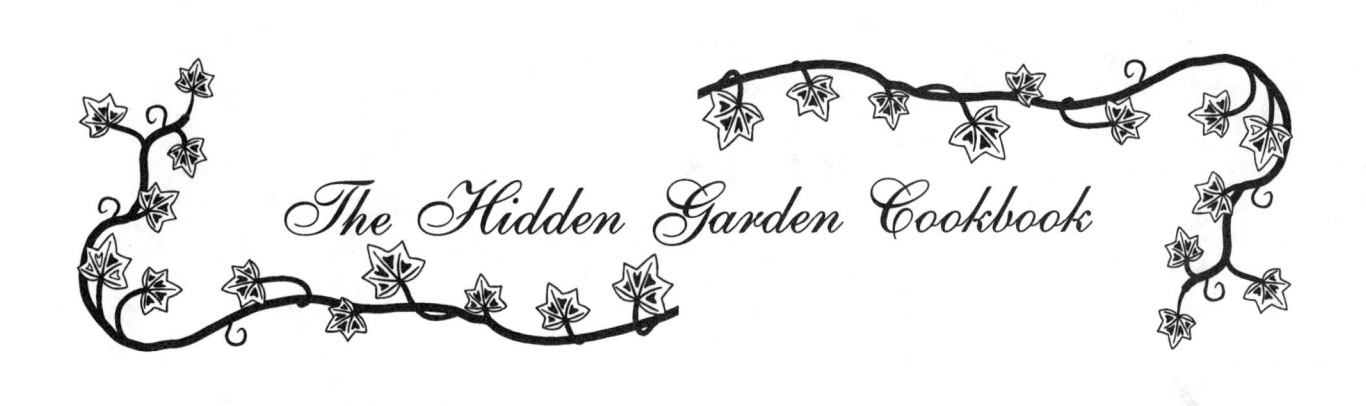

Desserts
&
Sweet Sauces

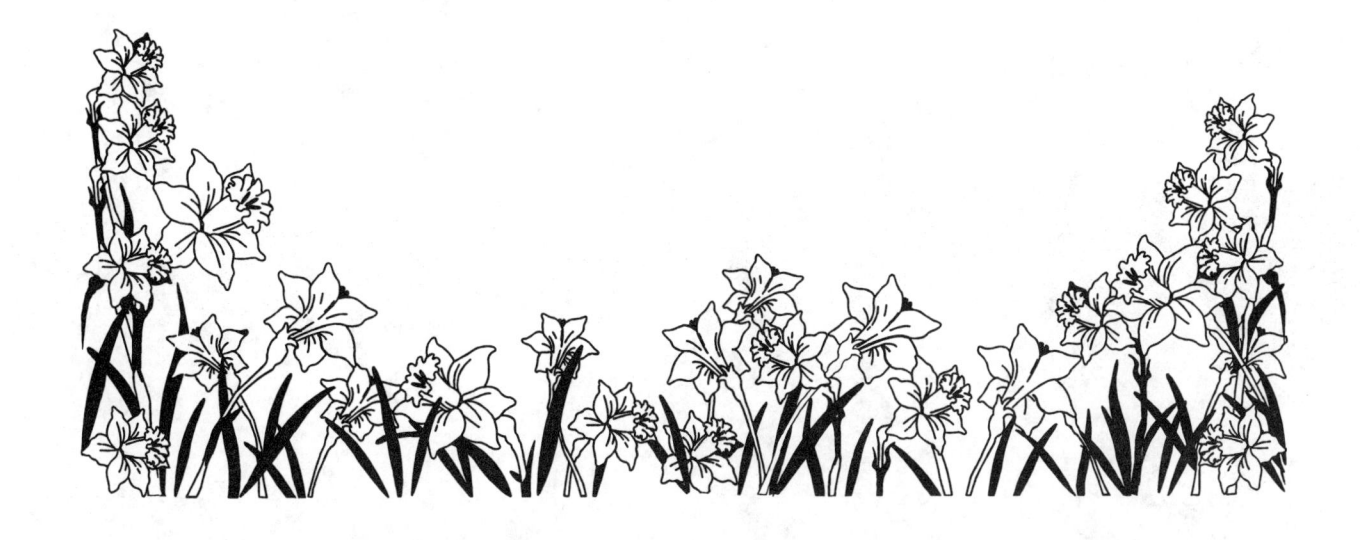

Poached Pears with Cinnamon Sticks

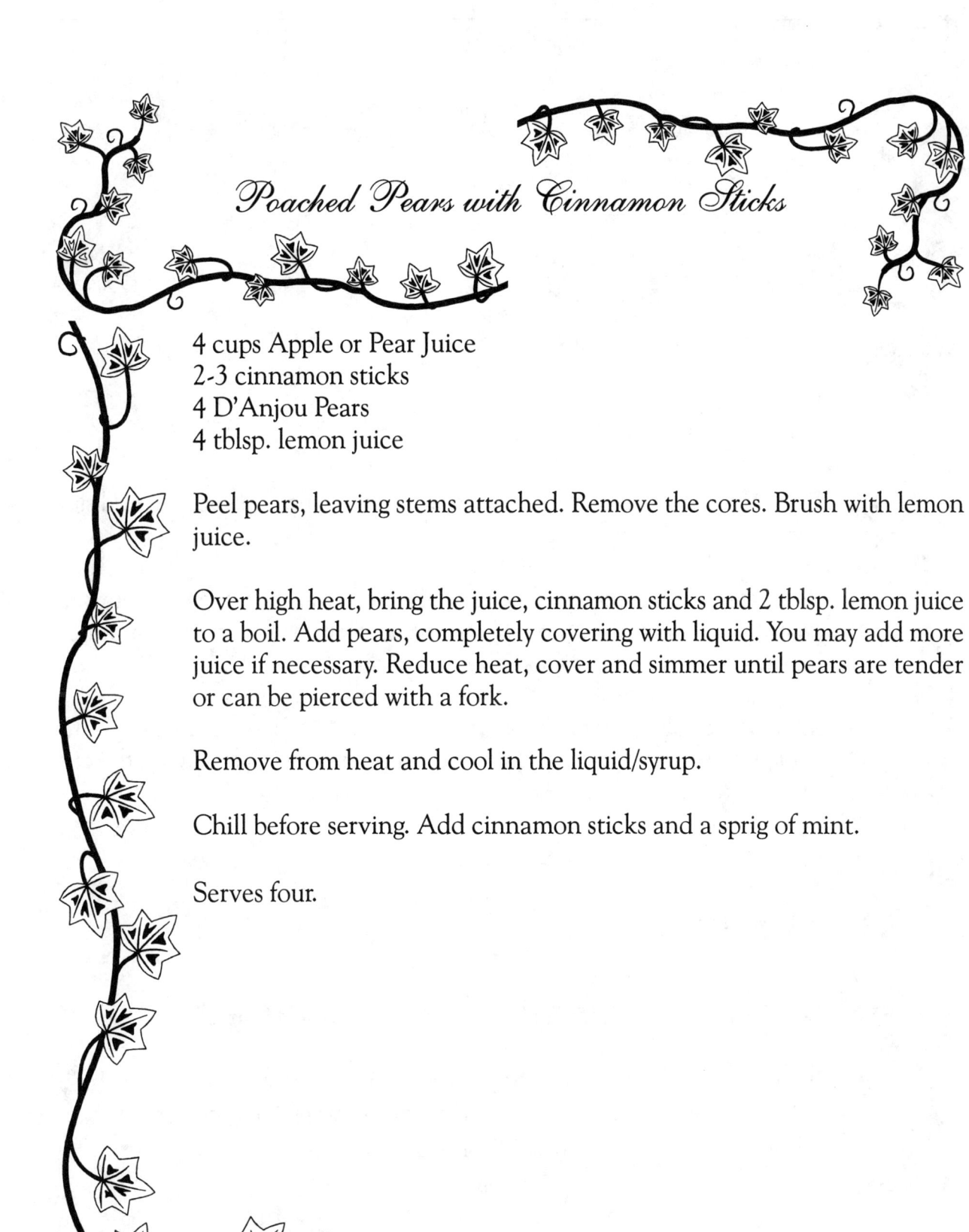

4 cups Apple or Pear Juice
2-3 cinnamon sticks
4 D'Anjou Pears
4 tblsp. lemon juice

Peel pears, leaving stems attached. Remove the cores. Brush with lemon juice.

Over high heat, bring the juice, cinnamon sticks and 2 tblsp. lemon juice to a boil. Add pears, completely covering with liquid. You may add more juice if necessary. Reduce heat, cover and simmer until pears are tender or can be pierced with a fork.

Remove from heat and cool in the liquid/syrup.

Chill before serving. Add cinnamon sticks and a sprig of mint.

Serves four.

Mother's Egg Custard

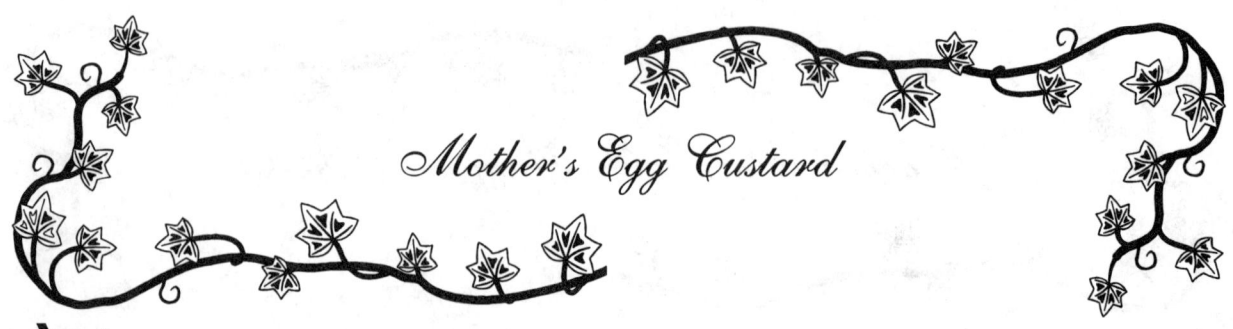

8 medium or 6 large eggs
3 cups lowfat milk
¼ cup sugar
1 tblsp. vanilla or white vanilla

Preheat the oven to 325°. Put 3 cups of milk in a heavy saucepan and simmer over medium heat while stirring continuously.

Beat eggs at high speed for 5-minutes, slowly adding sugar. Continue beating at medium speed until soft peaks form or for about 7-minutes. Mix warm milk, eggs and vanilla.

Meanwhile, place eight-baking cups in a baking pan with warm water enough to reach halfway up the baking cups. Fill baking cups with the custard mixture.

Bake for 30-40 minutes. Serve warm.

Serves eight.

Nola's Note: This makes a delicious Custard Sauce*.

If you can find "white" vanilla at your market, use it. The custard has a creamier appearance. The eggs and sugar in this recipe have already been reduced but you need to use whole eggs.

Poached Prunes and Apricot Compote

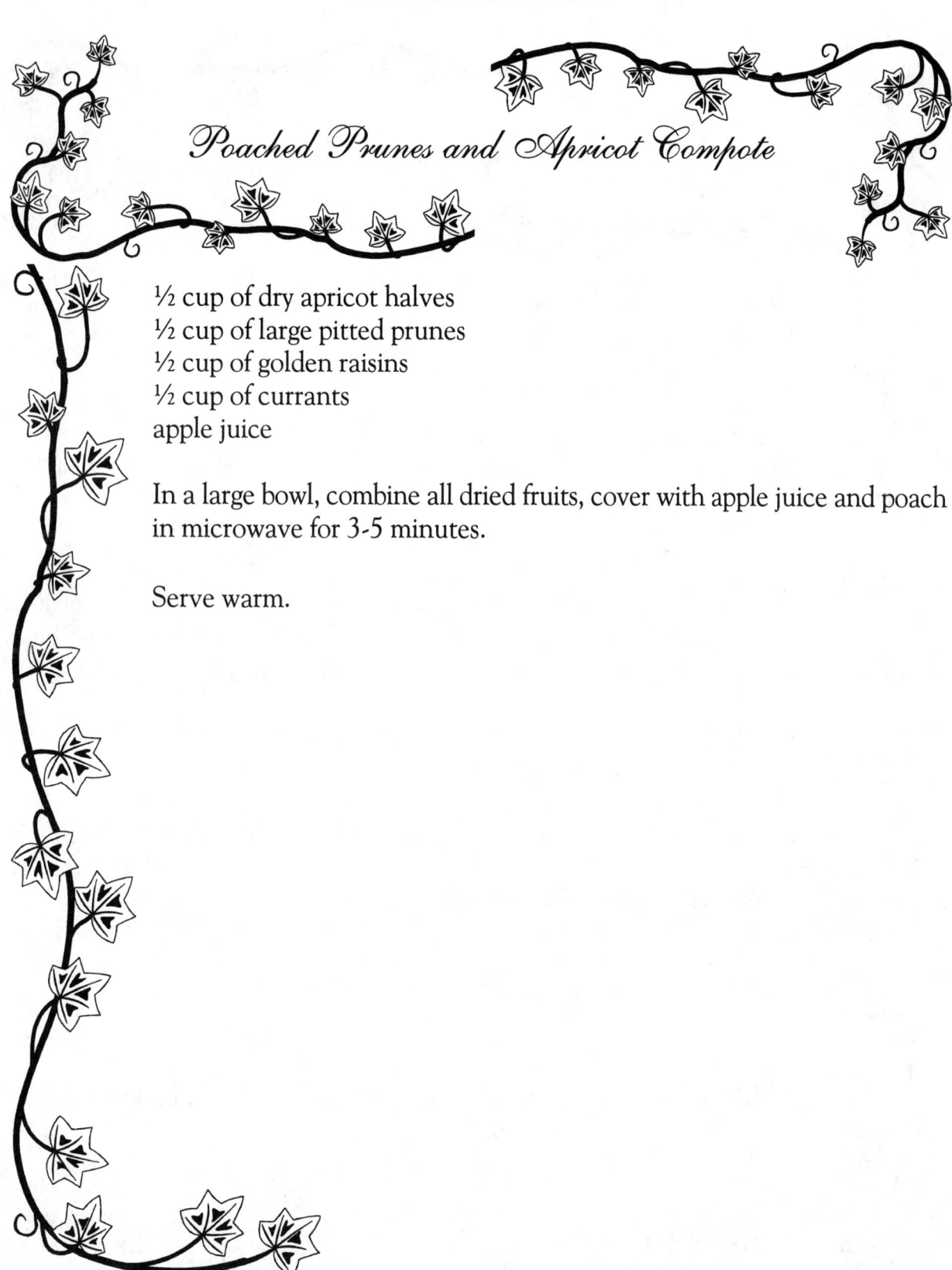

½ cup of dry apricot halves
½ cup of large pitted prunes
½ cup of golden raisins
½ cup of currants
apple juice

In a large bowl, combine all dried fruits, cover with apple juice and poach in microwave for 3-5 minutes.

Serve warm.

Yummy Tapioca Pudding

⅓ cup small pearl Tapioca
1½ cups Evaporated Milk
1½ cups lowfat milk
¼ cup sugar
2 eggs, well-beaten or 4 egg whites
3 tsp. vanilla or white vanilla

Pre-soak Tapioca in a bowl of cold water for 2-3 hours.

Strain well and put into a heavy pan with evaporated and lowfat milk and sugar. Cook over medium heat. Stir until boiling. Remove from heat. Slowly add beaten eggs while stirring continuously to avoid curdling.

Return to stove and over low heat, continue to cook while stirring until it achieves pudding consistency.

Let cool for 30-minutes before adding vanilla. Stir well and refrigerate.

Serve cold or warm. Garnish with a mint leaf or whole strawberry and a cookie.

Serves six.

Nola's Note: Here again, "white" vanilla gives the pudding a pure and elegant look.

Custard Sauce

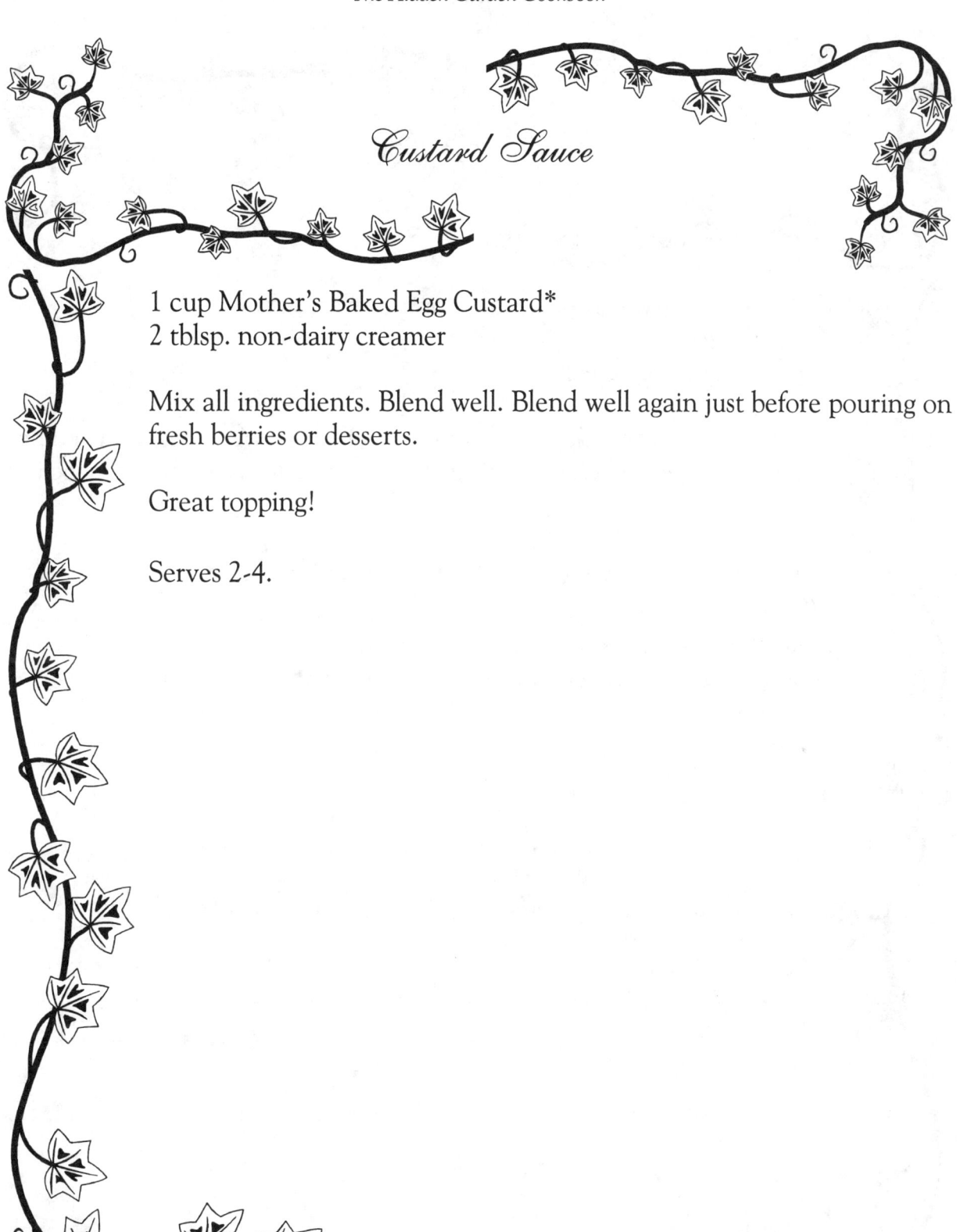

1 cup Mother's Baked Egg Custard*
2 tblsp. non-dairy creamer

Mix all ingredients. Blend well. Blend well again just before pouring on fresh berries or desserts.

Great topping!

Serves 2-4.

Creme Fraiche

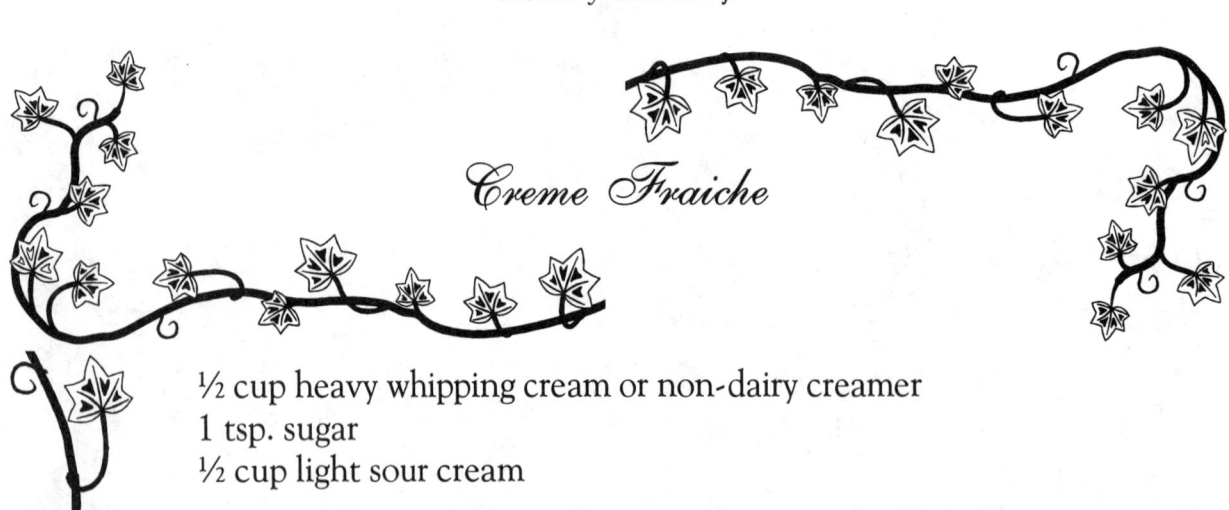

½ cup heavy whipping cream or non-dairy creamer
1 tsp. sugar
½ cup light sour cream

Mix heavy cream and light sour cream. Beat at low speed while adding sugar. Beat again before pouring on Chocolate Mousse, fresh blueberries or fresh raspberries.

Serves eight to ten—or less! Everyone will want seconds!

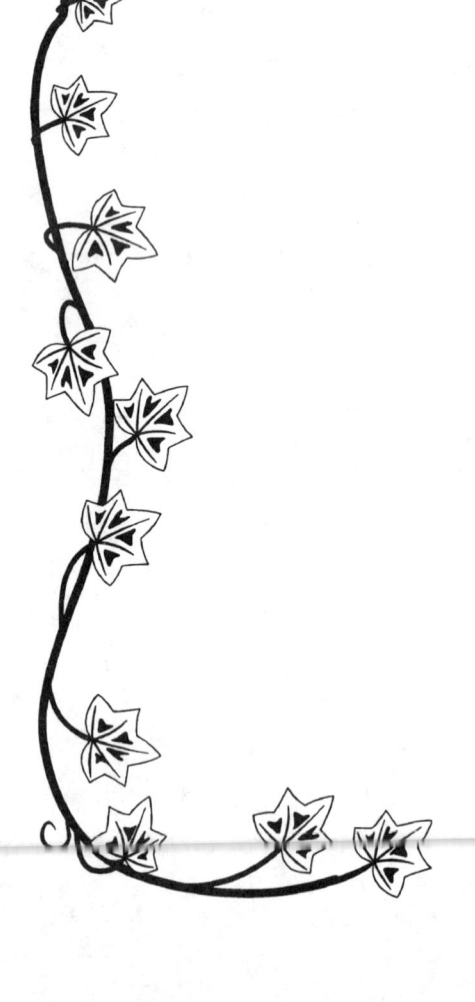

Footnotes

[1] *How to Choose a Qualified Plastic Surgeon* by the American Society of Plastic and Reconstructive Surgeons, Inc. Copyright 1989. Located: 444 E. Algonquin Rd., Arlington Heights, Illinois 60005 (1-800-635-0635)

[2] American Academy of Facial Plastic and Reconstructive Surgeons (AAFPRS), 1101 Vermont Avenue, N.W., Suite 404, Washington, D.C. 20005. (202) 842-4500.

[3] Lawrence Seifert, M.D., on the Board at UCLA and in private practice.

[4] *Clinics in Plastic Surgery* - Vol. 10, No. 4, October, 1983. Division of Plastic Surgery, Ohio State University, Symposium on Historical Perspectives of Plastic Surgery, "Plastic Surgery in the late 1920's" by Judith B. Zacher, M.D.

[5] Frank Ryan, M.D., elected to the UCLA Plastic Surgery Fellowship program and currently in private practice in Beverly Hills.

[6] Frank H. Ryan, M.D., is a plastic and reconstructive surgeon in Beverly Hills specializing in cosmetic surgery.

[7] *The Making of a Beautiful Face*, by J. Howard Crum, M.D., published in 1928.

[8] *Bottom Line*/Personal interview: "Wealth is Much More than Money by Jolton Roger and Peter McWilliams."

[9] *Health Confidential* interviewed Robin A.J. Youngson, MD, a Fellow in England's Royal College of Anaesthetists and currently staff anesthesiologist at Auckland Public Hospital, Auckland, New Zealand. Dr. Youngson is the author of *Operation! A Handbook for Surgical Patients*, David & Charles PLC, Brunel House, Newton Abbot, Devon, England.

[10] Williams, John, M.D., FACS.

[11] A Consumers Guide to Plastic Surgery/California Society of Plastic Surgeon.

[12] The Beverly Hills Institute of Aesthetic & Reconstructive Surgery, 416 N. Bedford Drive, Suite 200, Beverly Hills, California; (310) 278-8823.

[13] BIOMEDIC Clinical Care 1-800-66MEDIC for information and doctor in your area.

[14] John Williams, M.D., Museum Square, Los Angeles, California (213) 935-3644.

[15] Michael Churukian, M.D., Beverly Hills, California (310) 550-1545.

[16] Adrianna Scheibner, M.D., Beverly Hills, California (310) 274-1878.

[17] Sheila May, Licensed Medical Tatoo Artist, (310) 459-8090.

[18] Frank Ryan, M.D., Beverly Hills, California (310) 275-1075.

[19] Robert W. Hutcherson, M.D., Beverly Hills, California (310) 276-7012

[20] *Let's Develop!*, Dr. Fred Newman with Dr. Phyllis Goldberg.